Advances in Prevention and Management of Celiac Disease

Advances in Prevention and Management of Celiac Disease

Guest Editors

Maria Teresa Nestares Pleguezuelo
Rafael Martín-Masot

MDPI

Basel • Beijing • Wuhan • Barcelona • Belgrade • Novi Sad • Cluj • Manchester

Guest Editors
Maria Teresa Nestares Pleguezuelo
Dept Physiology
University of Granada
Granada
Spain

Rafael Martín-Masot
Pediatric Gastroenterology and Nutrition Unit
Hospital Regional Universitario de Malaga
Málaga
Spain

Editorial Office
MDPI AG
Grosspeteranlage 5
4052 Basel, Switzerland

This is a reprint of the Special Issue, published open access by the journal *Nutrients* (ISSN 2072-6643), freely accessible at: https://www.mdpi.com/journal/nutrients/special_issues/0XCTQNT183.

For citation purposes, cite each article independently as indicated on the article page online and as indicated below:

Lastname, A.A.; Lastname, B.B. Article Title. *Journal Name* **Year**, *Volume Number*, Page Range.

ISBN 978-3-7258-6334-1 (Hbk)
ISBN 978-3-7258-6335-8 (PDF)
https://doi.org/10.3390/books978-3-7258-6335-8

Contents

About the Editors

Maria Teresa Nestares Pleguezuelo

Teresa Nestares is a Full Professor of Physiology at the University of Granada, Spain, and a member of the Institute of Nutrition and Food Technology "José Mataix" (INYTA) at the Biomedical Research Centre (CIBM) of the University of Granada. Her research focuses on the relationship between diet and disease, particularly in cancer, celiac disease, and cardiovascular disorders. She has served as the principal investigator of several research projects, including those funded by the Regional Government of Andalusia, and has participated in over 30 funded research projects and contracts.

Prof. Nestares has published more than 100 scientific papers—half of them in first-quartile journals—and has an h-index of 21 (Web of Science). She has supervised 12 doctoral theses, has been an invited speaker at national and international conferences, and has served on the scientific committees of national congresses. In addition, she has acted as the Guest Editor for two Special Issues of *Nutrients* and currently coordinates the Official Master's Degree in Human Nutrition at the University of Granada. Her academic career has been recognized with multiple research and teaching awards, including the Extraordinary Doctoral Thesis Award.

Rafael Martín-Masot

Rafael Martín-Masot is a pediatric gastroenterologist at the Regional University Hospital of Málaga and Professor at the Department of Pharmacology and Pediatrics, Faculty of Medicine, University of Málaga, Spain. His research focuses on pediatric celiac disease, intestinal inflammation, and nutritional disorders. He has coordinated and participated in national and international research projects exploring body composition, gut microbiota, and omics-based biomarkers in gluten-related disorders. Dr. Martín-Masot has authored multiple peer-reviewed publications and book chapters, and serves as a reviewer for leading journals in pediatric gastroenterology and nutrition. He is also actively involved in teaching innovation and mentorship within undergraduate and postgraduate medical education.

nutrients

MDPI

Editorial

Advances in the Prevention and Management of Celiac Disease

Teresa Nestares [1,*] and Rafael Martín-Masot [2,3]

1 Department of Physiology, Faculty of Pharmacy, University of Granada, 18071 Granada, Spain
2 Pediatric Gastroenterology and Nutrition Unit, Hospital Regional Universitario de Malaga, 29010 Málaga, Spain; rafammgr@gmail.com
3 Department of Pharmacology and Pediatrics, School of Medicine, University of Málaga, 29010 Málaga, Spain
* Correspondence: nestares@ugr.es

Celiac disease (CD) exemplifies the complexity inherent in multifactorial, immune-mediated disorders, with layers of pathogenesis and clinical expression that continue to challenge both researchers and clinicians. Rather than a straightforward food intolerance, CD is now recognized as a systemic autoimmune disease with a heterogeneous clinical spectrum, capable of affecting any organ system and manifesting in both gastrointestinal and extraintestinal symptoms [1,2]. Over recent decades, the global prevalence of CD has steadily increased, accompanied by growing awareness of its diagnostic challenges, a broadening range of comorbidities, and the persistent need for improved strategies in both prevention and management [3,4].

Central to current research is the recognition that while gluten exposure is essential for the development of CD, it acts within a complex network of genetic and environmental factors [5]. Genetic predisposition—particularly HLA-DQ2 and DQ8—remains a fundamental requirement, yet disease susceptibility and clinical course are shaped by additional elements such as the timing and quantity of gluten introduction, the gut microbiota composition, dietary patterns, infectious exposures, impairment of the intestinal barrier, and maladaptive immune responses [6–10]. This intricate interplay highlights the urgency of refining our understanding of disease mechanisms, enhancing diagnostic accuracy, and developing innovative management strategies that extend beyond the gluten-free diet (GFD).

This Special Issue of *Nutrients* brings together eight original research articles and reviews that reflect the current State of the Art in CD, with a particular focus on environmental determinants and the ongoing search for novel preventive and therapeutic approaches. The collection includes comprehensive analyses of public health interventions and policy, such as a multicentric evaluation of how policies for celiac disease can transform patient lives across diverse settings (Contribution 1), and a nationwide assessment of eating attitudes and disordered eating risk in adults with CD in Brazil (Contribution 2). The nutritional landscape is further explored in pediatric and adolescent populations, with a comparative study of breakfast quality and the role of gluten-free products among Spanish children with and without CD (Contribution 3), as well as an investigation into the importance of early nutritional evaluation following the initiation of a GFD in children (Contribution 4).

Diagnostic innovation and monitoring are at the forefront in this issue, exemplified by the development and validation of a novel automated immunoassay for urinary immunogenic gluten peptides as a marker of dietary adherence (Contribution 5). The spectrum of clinical presentation is addressed in a large multicenter case–control study exploring the clinical, serological, and genetic differences between symptomatic and asymptomatic patients, raising important questions about current risk-based screening strategies (Contribution 6). The extraintestinal manifestations of CD are also considered, with a narrative

 https://doi.org/10.3390/nu17132240

review on the impact of gluten and CD on male and female reproductive health (Contribution 7), expanding our perspective on the systemic effects of the disease.

Finally, the Special Issue underscores the transformative potential of omics sciences—particularly metabolomics—in CD research and clinical care. A State-of-the-Art review explores how metabolomic profiling is shedding light on early diagnosis, disease monitoring, and the molecular impact of the GFD, pointing toward a future of precision medicine and targeted interventions (Contribution 8).

Together, these contributions highlight the necessity of a multidisciplinary, evidence-based, and technologically advanced approach to CD. The future of research and clinical care in CD will depend on collaboration among clinicians, nutritionists, molecular scientists, and data specialists, all working to translate molecular insights into meaningful patient outcomes.

We are deeply grateful to all authors, reviewers, and the editorial staff at *Nutrients* for their dedication to this Special Issue. It is our hope that the research presented here will foster further innovation, inspire new collaborations, and ultimately advance the care and quality of life of all individuals living with CD.

Author Contributions: T.N. and R.M.-M. edited the manuscript. All authors have read and agreed to the published version of the manuscript.

Funding: No funding was received for the production of this Editorial.

Conflicts of Interest: The authors declare no conflicts of interest.

List of Contributions

1. Falcomer, A.L.; Pratesi, C.B.; Nakano, E.Y.; Chaves, C.; Rostami-Nejad, M.; Guennouni, M.; Aksan, A.; Pouchot, J.; Häuser, W.; Zandonadi, R.P. From Struggle to Strength: A Multi-centric Study on How Public Policies for Celiac Disease Transform Lives. *Nutrients* **2024**, *16*, 2855. https://doi.org/10.3390/nu16172855.
2. Franco, L.; Nakano, E.Y.; Raposo, A.; Alturki, H.A.; Alarifi, S.N.; Chaves, C.; Teixeira-Lemos, E.; Romão, B. Eating Attitudes of Patients with Celiac Disease in Brazil: A Nationwide Assessment with the EAT-26 Instrument. *Nutrients* **2023**, *15*, 4796. https://doi.org/10.3390/nu15224796.
3. Úbeda, N.; González, M.P.; Achón, M.; García-González, Á.; Ballestero-Fernández, C.; Fajardo, V.; Alonso-Aperte, E. Nutritional Composition of Breakfast in Children and Adolescents with and without Celiac Disease in Spain—Role of Gluten-Free Commercial Products. *Nutrients* **2023**, *15*, 2368. https://doi.org/10.3390/nu15102368.
4. Martín-Masot, R.; Jiménez-Muñoz, M.; Herrador-López, M.; Flor-Alemany, M.; Navas-López, V.M.; Nestares, T. The Importance of an Early Evaluation after Establishing a Gluten-Free Diet in Children with Celiac Disease. *Nutrients* **2023**, *15*, 1761. https://doi.org/10.3390/nu15071761.
5. Segura, V.; Ruiz-Carnicer, Á.; Mendía, I.; Garzón-Benavides, M.; Pizarro, Á.E.; Comino, I.; Sousa, C. Evaluation of the Usefulness of an Automatable Immunoassay for Monitoring Celiac Disease by Quantification of Immunogenic Gluten Peptides in Urine. *Nutrients* **2023**, *15*, 1730. https://doi.org/10.3390/nu15071730.
6. Castillejo, G.; Ochoa-Sangrador, C.; Pérez-Solís, D.; Cilleruelo, M.L.; Donat, E.; García-Burriel, J.I.; Sánchez-Valverde, F.; Garcia-Calatayud, S.; Eizaguirre, F.J.; Martinez-Ojinaga, E.; et al. Coeliac Disease Case–Control Study: Has the Time Come to Explore beyond Patients at Risk? *Nutrients* **2023**, *15*, 1267. https://doi.org/10.3390/nu15051267.
7. Wieser, H.; Ciacci, C.; Soldaini, C.; Gizzi, C.; Pellegrini, L.; Santonicola, A. Fertility in Celiac Disease: The Impact of Gluten on Male and Female Reproductive Health. *Nutrients* **2025**, *17*, 1575. https://doi.org/10.3390/nu17091575.

8. Martín-Masot, R.; Jiménez-Muñoz, M.; Herrador-López, M.; Navas-López, V.M.; Obis, E.; Jové, M.; Pamplona, R.; Nestares, T. Metabolomic Profiling in Children with Celiac Disease: Beyond the Gluten-Free Diet. *Nutrients* **2023**, *15*, 2871. https://doi.org/10.3390/nu15132871.

References

1. Husby, S.; Koletzko, S.; Korponay-Szabó, I.; Kurppa, K.; Mearin, M.L.; Ribes-Koninckx, C.; Shamir, R.; Troncone, R.; Auricchio, R.; Castillejo, G.; et al. European Society Paediatric Gastroenterology, Hepatology and Nutrition Guidelines for Diagnosing Coeliac Disease 2020. *J. Pediatr. Gastroenterol. Nutr.* **2020**, *70*, 141–156. [CrossRef] [PubMed]
2. Catassi, C.; Verdu, E.F.; Bai, J.C.; Lionetti, E. Coeliac disease. *Lancet* **2022**, *399*, 2413–2426. [CrossRef] [PubMed]
3. King, J.A.; Jeong, J.; Underwood, F.E.; Quan, J.; Panaccione, N.; Windsor, J.W.; Coward, S.; deBruyn, J.; Ronksley, P.E.; Shaheen, A.-A.; et al. Incidence of Celiac Disease Is Increasing Over Time: A Systematic Review and Meta-Analysis. *Am. J. Gastroenterol.* **2020**, *115*, 507–525. [CrossRef] [PubMed]
4. Mearin, M.L.; Agardh, D.; Antunes, H.; Al-Toma, A.; Auricchio, R.; Castillejo, G.; Catassi, C.; Ciacci, C.; Discepolo, V.; Dolinsek, J.; et al. ESPGHAN Position Paper on Management and Follow-up of Children and Adolescents With Celiac Disease. *J. Pediatr. Gastroenterol. Nutr.* **2022**, *75*, 369–386. [CrossRef] [PubMed]
5. Iversen, R.; Sollid, L.M. The Immunobiology and Pathogenesis of Celiac Disease. *Annu. Rev. Pathol.* **2023**, *18*, 47–70. [CrossRef] [PubMed]
6. Silvester, J.A.; Comino, I.; Rigaux, L.N.; Segura, V.; Green, K.H.; Cebolla, A.; Weiten, D.; Dominguez, R.; Leffler, D.A.; Leon, F.; et al. Exposure sources, amounts and time course of gluten ingestion and excretion in patients with coeliac disease on a gluten-free diet. *Aliment. Pharmacol. Ther.* **2020**, *52*, 1469–1479. [CrossRef] [PubMed]
7. Akobeng, A.K.; Singh, P.; Kumar, M.; Al Khodor, S. Role of the gut microbiota in the pathogenesis of coeliac disease and potential therapeutic implications 2020. *Eur. J. Nutr.* **2020**, *59*, 3369–3390. [CrossRef] [PubMed]
8. De Re, V.; Magris, R.; Cannizzaro, R. New Insights into the Pathogenesis of Celiac Disease. *Front. Med.* **2017**, *4*, 137. [CrossRef] [PubMed]
9. Dubois, P.C.; van Heel, D.A. Translational mini-review series on the immunogenetics of gut disease: Immunogenetics of coeliac disease. *Clin. Exp. Immunol.* **2008**, *153*, 162–173. [CrossRef] [PubMed]
10. Zingone, F.; Bai, J.C.; Cellier, C.; Ludvigsson, J.F. Celiac Disease-Related Conditions: Who to Test? *Gastroenterology* **2024**, *167*, 64–78. [CrossRef] [PubMed]

nutrients MDPI

Review

Metabolomic Profiling in Children with Celiac Disease: Beyond the Gluten-Free Diet

Rafael Martín-Masot [1,2], María Jiménez-Muñoz [1,*], Marta Herrador-López [1], Víctor Manuel Navas-López [1], Elia Obis [3], Mariona Jové [3], Reinald Pamplona [3] and Teresa Nestares [2,4]

1 Pediatric Gastroenterology and Nutrition Unit, Hospital Regional Universitario de Malaga, 29010 Málaga, Spain; rafammgr@gmail.com (R.M.-M.); herradorlopezm@gmail.com (M.H.-L.); victor.navas@gmail.com (V.M.N.-L.)
2 Institute of Nutrition and Food Technology "José MataixVerdú" (INYTA), Biomedical Research Centre (CIBM), University of Granada, 18071 Granada, Spain; nestares@ugr.es
3 Department of Experimental Medicine, Lleida Biomedical Research Institute (IRBLleida), University of Lleida (UdL), 25198 Lleida, Spain; eobis@irblleida.cat (E.O.); mariona.jove@udl.cat (M.J.); reinald.pamplona@udl.cat (R.P.)
4 Department of Physiology, Faculty of Pharmacy, University of Granada, 18071 Granada, Spain
* Correspondence: mariajmnzm@gmail.com; Tel.: +34-686167643

Abstract: Celiac disease (CD) is included in the group of complex or multifactorial diseases, i.e., those caused by the interaction of genetic and environmental factors. Despite a growing understanding of the pathophysiological mechanisms of the disease, diagnosis is still often delayed and there are no effective biomarkers for early diagnosis. The only current treatment, a gluten-free diet (GFD), can alleviate symptoms and restore intestinal villi, but its cellular effects remain poorly understood. To gain a comprehensive understanding of CD's progression, it is crucial to advance knowledge across various scientific disciplines and explore what transpires after disease onset. Metabolomics studies hold particular significance in unravelling the complexities of multifactorial and multisystemic disorders, where environmental factors play a significant role in disease manifestation and progression. By analyzing metabolites, we can gain insights into the reasons behind CD's occurrence, as well as better comprehend the impact of treatment initiation on patients. In this review, we present a collection of articles that showcase the latest breakthroughs in the field of metabolomics in pediatric CD, with the aim of trying to identify CD biomarkers for both early diagnosis and treatment monitoring. These advancements shed light on the potential of metabolomic analysis in enhancing our understanding of the disease and improving diagnostic and therapeutic strategies. More studies need to be designed to cover metabolic profiles in subjects at risk of developing the disease, as well as those analyzing biomarkers for follow-up treatment with a GFD.

Keywords: celiac disease; gluten-free diet; metabolomics; children; immune; intestinal

1. Introduction

Celiac disease (CD) is included in the group of complex or multifactorial diseases, i.e., those caused by the interaction of genetic and environmental factors [1]. It is a chronic disease whose severity and digestive and/or systemic symptoms show great variability among patients. However, the common characteristic to all of them is an exacerbated immune response to gluten and related proteins, so this systemic disorder is considered an immune-mediated disease. In fact, patients are characterized by the presence of high titers of specific antibodies and the vast majority are carriers of the DQ2 and/or DQ8 haplotypes of the major histocompatibility complex (Human Leukocyte Antigen, HLA class II), responsible for antigen presentation by the immune system [2–4]. In addition to gluten intake and the presence of risk alleles in HLA, the occurrence of intestinal and extra-intestinal symptoms in CD requires the activation of both types of immune response, innate and adaptive, and this overactivation of the immune system is observed at the intestinal level as well as at the peripheral and systemic levels [4].

The main gap in the knowledge of the pathogenesis of CD is an explanation of why 25–35% of the world's healthy population has these haplotypes, but only about 1–3% will develop CD [5,6]. It is possible that other environmental and genetic factors influence an individual's ability to induce and control the innate response and an individual's susceptibility to gluten.

Even though CD is actually one of the most frequent genetic diseases, affecting 1–3% of the world's population, and to a greater extent women and children [7], it is clearly underestimated and underdiagnosed. Despite advances in knowledge and the development of serological tests, CD continues to be difficult and costly to diagnose, largely due to the systemic nature of CD, the lack of specificity of its clinical manifestations and the existence of silent or latent forms [8,9]. The problem is that untreated celiacs or those whose diagnosis has been delayed, despite having no symptoms, may have an exacerbated and chronic activation of the immune system, which is uncontrolled for a longer time, leading to a worse prognosis, an accentuation of symptoms and the appearance of other autoimmune diseases such as type 1 diabetes or gluten-dependent hepatitis, which are frequent in CD patients [10,11]. Also, they may be affected by a variety of adverse consequences, some serious such as the development of malignant tumors [12]. Therefore, at the present time, the main challenge, like for other genetic-based diseases (such as some types of cancer and diabetes, among others), is to study in genetically predisposed individuals, on the one hand, which factors are involved in the development or not of CD and, on the other, to find biomarkers for its early diagnosis and follow-up. The idea is to avoid the side effects when the disease has already made its debut and even prevent its appearance, something relevant since it is currently incurable.

The only current treatment for CD is a lifelong strict gluten-free diet (GFD) that achieves a remission of symptoms within a few days or weeks and a restoration of intestinal villi and immune homeostasis within a few months. We ourselves have found that, after 18 months of a strict GFD follow-up, the celiac has most of the parameters equivalent to those of a healthy child [13–15]. This is an important finding, but, even so, the usual delay in diagnosis (because of its difficulty), in combination with the time it takes to stabilize the disease, is too long, and in this period they may develop complications that will result in sequelae that range from minor (e.g., permanent short stature, dental enamel failure and psychiatric problems) to serious, such as tumors, in the long term. The fact is that the GFD seems to play an important role in the pathogenesis of tumor development, since some studies have described a greater development of tumors the later the diagnosis is made and in patients who have not followed the GFD [16]. Thus, untreated CD is associated above all with T-cell lymphoma (EATL) [12] and small bowel adenocarcinoma [17], although a higher incidence of non-Hodgkin's lymphoma and colorectal cancer has also been described [18,19].

As CD is a systemic and complex disease, it is necessary to look at it from different perspectives. Personalized or precision medicine refers to the application of biotechnology, genetic profiling, "omics" sciences and the incorporation of clinical and environmental factors to evaluate individual risks and design strategies for the prevention, diagnosis, treatment or follow-up of the disease at the right time and in the right patient, with the minimum toxicity and maximum possible efficacy. One of the sciences that has been booming in recent years is metabolomics, which deals with the study of chemical processes in which small molecules, called metabolites, which can be both endogenous and xenobiotic, are measured. These molecules give information about a metabolic process that has taken place in the organism, and metabolomics can be considered, from this perspective, as an approach to cellular metabolism that other "omics" sciences cannot provide [20,21]. In this sense, metabolomics is presented as a fast and non-invasive tool that could represent a step forward in the knowledge of many diseases through the study of the metabolic profile by obtaining what are known as "metabolomic fingerprints or signatures" resulting from the interaction of the genome, epigenome, transcriptome, proteome and the environment.

Metabolomics studies are especially relevant in those multifactorial and multisystemic pathological situations where the environmental factor plays a relevant role in the appearance and development of the disease. Technologies such as metabolomics could define the alterations that occur in the genetically predisposed individual, as well as after certain changes, such as the GFD, helping to better understand these complex interactions, and thus may be useful for the diagnosis and monitoring of CD [22]. In this review, we cover several articles highlighting the latest advancements in the field of metabolomics in pediatric CD. Specifically, we explore studies that examine plasma and urine samples, with a special focus on the role of the GFD.

The main objective of this work was to compile the results of recent studies on the metabolomic profile of pediatric celiac patients, both at diagnosis and throughout the establishment of the GFD and the evolution of the disease, as well as its comparison with healthy children with/without genetic risk of CD. The ultimate objective was to establish the foundations of current knowledge on the subject, enabling the development of future research, ideally with the creation of new biomarkers. These biomarkers would facilitate an optimized management of the disease beyond the GFD.

2. Materials and Methods

We obtained published studies related to the topic in MEDLINE or PubMed, Scopus, Embase and Web of Science. The narrative review was conducted in March and April 2023. Search terms used were "metabolomics", "metabolome", "celiac/coeliac disease", "metabolites" "biomarkers", "gluten free diet". Filters applied were child: birth–18 years; infant: birth–23 months; infant: 1–23 months; newborn: birth–1 month; preschool child: 2–5 years; child: 6–12 years; adolescent: 13–18 years. Articles published in English or Spanish were selected for critical synthesis. We included studies carried out on blood (plasma/serum) and urine. The search was completed with a review of bibliographic references. Exclusion criteria included articles that lacked a comprehensive description of the study in their full texts, studies published in non-peer-reviewed journals, meta-analyses, reviews, protocols, editorials and letters to the editor and studies conducted on animal models.

3. Metabolomics Platforms

Clinical metabolomics is a rising field of clinical research that takes advantage of the great technological advances that have been developed in recent years. This relatively new discipline involves the systematic analysis of metabolites (small molecules involved in metabolic pathways) in biological samples such as blood, urine and tissues to identify and measure the unique metabolic profile of an individual [23–25]. This profile can provide valuable information about an individual's health status, including disease diagnosis, prognosis and treatment response [26–28]. Clinical metabolomics integrates various analytical techniques, such as mass spectrometry (MS) and nuclear magnetic resonance (NMR) spectroscopy, to detect and quantify metabolites in biological samples [29–31]. The data obtained from metabolomic analysis can be used to develop personalized and precision medicine strategies, by identifying biomarkers and metabolic pathways associated with specific diseases or conditions [32].

Clinical metabolomics is of great importance in medical and biomedical research because it allows the identification of metabolic biomarkers that can be used for the early detection, diagnosis and monitoring of diseases [30]. By analyzing changes in metabolic profiles, clues can be obtained about the pathogenesis of diseases and the underlying molecular mechanisms [31,33–39]. Using this technique allows the scientific and clinical community to follow and evaluate a wide variety of physiological conditions, such as the physiological changes that occur during pregnancy or aging [40–43] as well as for the diagnosis and monitoring of different diseases such as diabetes, cancer or neurodegenerative diseases [44–50]. In addition, clinical metabolomics can also help to develop new drugs and improve the efficacy and safety of existing treatments by providing information on how patients metabolize and respond to drugs [51–54]. It has the potential to improve diagnostic accuracy, treatment efficacy and understanding of the biological mechanisms underlying diseases [55].

The two most common techniques used in data acquisition for metabolomics analyses are NMR and MS [55]. Table 1 shows some of the key differences between the two techniques [47,56–60]. The principle of NMR spectroscopy is based on the interaction between the magnetic moments of atomic nuclei and an external magnetic field [61,62]. When a sample is placed in a magnetic field and irradiated with radiofrequency energy, the nuclei absorb and re-emit energy at characteristic frequencies, which is used to obtain information about the chemical environment and structure of the molecules. In the case of clinical metabolomics, NMR spectroscopy is used to analyze biological samples containing a complex mixture of metabolites [29]. The sample is prepared by extracting the metabolites and dissolving them in a deuterated solvent to prevent interference from the solvent itself. The sample is then placed in an NMR spectrometer, where it is subjected to a strong magnetic field and radiofrequency energy [63].

Table 1. Key differences between clinical metabolomics platforms.

	Nuclear Magnetic Resonance (NMR)	Mass Spectrometry (MS)
Sensitivity	Low	High
Dynamic range	Moderate	High
Reproducibility	Very high	Moderate
Detectable metabolites	30–100	300–5000 or more
Metabolite identification	Well categorized	Labor intensive
Targeted analysis	Not optimal	Better than NMR
Sample destructive	Non-destructive	Destructive to sample
Sample preparation	Minimal	More complex than NMR
Tissue extraction	Not required	Required
Sample analysis time	Fast (<10 min)	Longer than NMR (>10 min)
Instrument cost	High	Cheaper than NMR
Sample cost	Low	High

Adapted from different authors [56–60].

MS is the other main technique used in clinical metabolomics to detect and quantify metabolites in biological samples such as blood, urine and tissues [64]. The principle of MS is based on the ionization of molecules and the separation of ions based on their mass-to-charge ratio (m/z) in a mass analyzer [65]. The sample is first ionized, usually by using an ionization source such as electrospray ionization (ESI), atmospheric pressure chemical ionization (APCI) or matrix-assisted laser desorption/ionization [66–70] (MALDI). The ions are then separated and detected by the mass analyzer, which produces a mass spectrum showing the abundance of ions at different m/z values. The sample is prepared by extracting the metabolites and separating them from other compounds that may interfere with the analysis. The extracted metabolites are then subjected to ionization and analyzed by MS. It can detect and quantify a wide range of metabolites with high sensitivity and specificity, making it a powerful tool for clinical metabolomics research [60]. In addition, MS can be coupled with chromatography techniques such as liquid chromatography (LC) or gas chromatography (GC), which allows for further separation and analysis of metabolites. This approach, known as LC-MS or GC-MS [71–73], is a common method used in clinical metabolomics to analyze complex samples [74]. The pitfalls of the technique are that sample processing is more complex and that costs per sample are higher than in NMR. However, MS is the technique that is used the most in clinical metabolomics research due to its ability to detect and quantify a wide range of metabolites with high sensitivity and specificity [58].

Both techniques, apart from using different detectors, also need appropriate sample processing according to the technique that will be used, as well as different data processing and analysis in each case [75]. Sample preparation is key in these analyses [60,76,77], as well as the selected approach for the experimental design, i.e., whether the metabolomic analysis is directed or not [29]. When we want to gain a global idea of the metabolic profile of a particular sample to open new questions or to see general changes, an untargeted analysis is used [43,78,79]. If we want to analyze only a more specific set of metabolites, which are usually related either by structure or by belonging to the same metabolic pathway, we use a targeted analysis [80,81]. In both cases, sample preparation and data analysis follow a slightly different workflow [82]. Figure 1 shows some of the key steps in clinical metabolomics approaches.

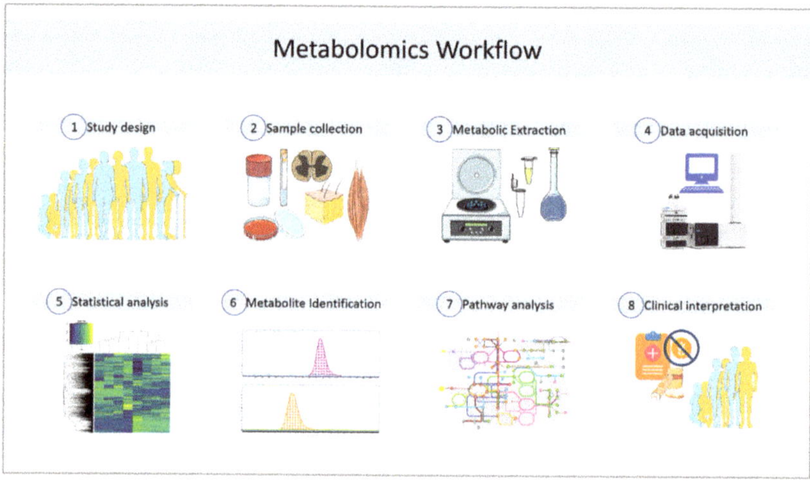

Figure 1. General workflow for clinical metabolomics studies. Author contributions. This figure was partly generated using Servier Medical Art, provided by Servier, licensed under a Creative Commons Attribution 3.0 unported license.

The clinical applications of metabolomics are many and diverse. Among them are the identification of biomarkers of diseases, the development of new therapies [28,83–85], the personalization of medical treatments [52,54], the early detection of diseases or the monitoring of the progression of diseases and response to treatment [86–89]. All of them have great value for the scientific and health community, as well as for all of society. In recent years, different technologies and methodologies for metabolomics have been developed and improved, which can help overcome some of the current challenges and enable significant advances in medical and biomedical research. Some of the new technologies and methodologies under development include ion mobility, metabolic flux analysis or separation-free MS techniques for direct infusion acquisition or metabolic imaging [90–101]. Although there are challenges in the implementation of clinical metabolomics, such as metabolite identification, the standardization of analysis techniques and the interpretation of complex data, new technologies and methodologies are constantly developing and can help overcome these barriers [29]. It is necessary to foster interdisciplinary collaboration to advance the field of clinical metabolomics, since the combination of knowledge and skills from different disciplines, such as biochemistry, bioinformatics, medicine and engineering, can lead to significant advances in the understanding of physiology and disease and in the development of personalized treatments.

4. Plasma Metabolomic Profile

4.1. CD's Inherent Footprint and Role of the GFD

Several molecules have been proposed as potential CD biomarkers. In this regard, Auricchio et al., 2019 [102] found that the serum phospholipid profile is different in children who develop CD compared to healthy children with similar genetic profiles (specific celiac human HLA DQ2 or DQ8), even before the introduction of gluten to the diet at 4 months of age. They followed a cohort of children from families with a CD case from birth to 8 years of age, with sampling at 4 and 12 months of age (and at CD diagnosis in cases >24 months of age), finding in lipidomic analysis based on LC coupled with MS and multiple reaction monitoring (MRM) that the lipid profile is fairly constant in each individual, in both groups, suggesting that it could be constitutive. In the age-grouped analysis, they found that children who developed CD had increased lyso- and phosphatidylcholine (PC) serum levels (PC 40:4 showed the greatest difference between the two groups), as well as alkylacylphosphatidylcholine (PC-O). Specifically, two alkylacylphosphatidylcholipids (PC O-42:0 and PC O-38:3), together with breastfeeding and one phosphatidylcholine (PC 34:1), were defined as predictors of CD development. They found that phosphatidylethanolamines (PE) PE 34:1 and PE 36:1 were decreased in celiac patients.

The working group of Sen et al., 2019 [103] also applied lipidomics in the study of a cohort of Finnish children in the context of the Type 1 Diabetes Prediction and Prevention study. Based on MS and comparing plasma samples from children who developed CD with plasma samples from healthy controls, matched for HLA risk, sex and age, they found that CD progressors (children who developed CD) had increased triacylgycerols (TGs) of low carbon number, double-bond count plasma levels and decreased phosphatidylcholines and cholesterol esters levels at 3 months of age compared to controls. These differences were not apparent at birth (cord blood) and exacerbated with age. It is proposed that the increase in TGs of low carbon number and double-bond count is due to de novo lipogenesis compensating for lipid malabsorption, which would occur at a very young age; this increase in TGs has been linked in adults to increased liver fat in non-alcoholic fatty liver disease [104]. In addition, they found decreased total essential TG levels in the plasma of the CD progressors after gluten intake, reversing this trend, but not significantly, after the onset of GFD, and there was an inverse relationship with the tissue transglutaminase IgA titer (tTGA). There was also an increase in cholesterol levels after the start of GFD in the CD progressors. On the other hand, the endogenous TGs plasma levels were decreased in CD progressors independently of gluten intake. PCs were elevated in both CD progressors and controls after the start of gluten intake. A difference in sphingomyelin plasma levels was observed in CD progressors at a later age, after the introduction of GFD.

These findings suggest that a dysregulation in lipid metabolism may be associated with the development of CD, and that it occurs in the first months of life, even before the introduction of gluten to the diet. This could help predict the development of CD in infants at genetic risk, even years before the appearance of specific antibodies or clinical symptoms/signs.

However, a previous study (2016) based on the PreventCD project suggested that the metabolic profile at 4 months (before the introduction of gluten to the diet) did not predict the development of CD, but that metabolic pathways are affected later in life [105]. In this study, which studied serum samples from infants at genetic risk for CD who developed CD compared to those who did not develop the disease at 8 years of age, a trend of decreased phospholipids levels was found in children who subsequently developed CD, although not significantly, with a greater decrease in the subsample of children exclusively breastfed until 4 months of age. They conclude that metabolomic studies should focus on children who have already had gluten introduced to their diet. However, this study focused the analysis on phospholipids and acylcarnitines, and TGs and cholesterol esters were not measured.

Following the lipidomics approach, in a pilot study conducted by ourselves [106], plasma lipid profile was affected in celiac patients, despite GFD treatment. Using an

LC-MS/MS platform, there plasma from 17 celiac children under a GFD treatment and 17 healthy controls (siblings) was analyzed. Among the significant molecules, it was found that 64% were increased and 36% decreased in CD patients. Two carboxylic acids and derivatives were increased in CD; other molecules whose levels were affected in patients were four fatty acyls (thromboxanes and leykotrienes involved in inflammatory pathways), five glycerolipids, eleven glycerophospholipids, one organoxigen compound and two sphingolipids, lipid species belonging to steroid metabolism and other molecules involved in bilirubin metabolism. In celiac patients elevated levels of molecules involved in cell signaling pathways (ceramides, diacylglycerides and lysophospholipids) were found. Diacylglycerides play a central role in the control of neuronal communication, phagocytosis and the control of immune responses, and as a second messenger they play an important role in the regulation of mTOR, recently described as a key factor in maintaining a sustained inflammatory response in CD [107].

Aside from the lipid profile, one-carbon metabolism alterations were also found by this group [108] under a targeted plasma metabolomics study. They observed a down-regulation of the trans-sulphuration pathway in CD patients, despite GFD, with decreased cysteine and cystathionine, which, together with normal glutathione and vitamin B6, suggests a specific defect at the level of the enzymes involved in antioxidant defense, oxygen sensing, mitochondrial function, inflammation and second-messenger signaling. This finding, moreover, could be explained by a S-adenosyl-L-homocysteine (SAH) hydrolase mutation that causes typical symptoms of the disease, such as growth retardation, dental anomalies or hypertransaminasemia. In contrast, other pathways involved in one-carbon metabolism appeared to be preserved (choline metabolism, the methionine cycle and the folate cycle), suggesting that adherence to a strict GFD could reverse certain metabolic changes in celiac patients, making them resemble the profile of healthy subjects. This group notes that these metabolomic changes are, however, minor, as only approximately 4% of the total plasma metabolome analyzed was affected [106].

In a more recent study based on a targeted plasma metabolomics analysis, Girdhar et al., 2023 [109] found increased levels of 2-methyl-3-ketovalric acid, taurodeoxycholic acid (TDCA), glucono-D-lactone and isoburyryl-L-carnitine, as well as significantly low oleic acid levels (anti-inflammatory metabolite) in CD progressors (compared to healthy children matched for age, HLA genotype, breastfeeding duration and gluten exposure duration). Other metabolic pathways were also affected in the CD progressors, such as the pentose phosphate pathway, unsaturated fatty acid biosynthesis and glycolipid and linoleic acid metabolism. Notably, TDCA levels were increased to twice the normal values. TDCA, a metabolite derived from the gut microbiota, may play a role in small intestinal inflammation and CD pathogenesis, as its administration to C57BL/6J mice by supplementing their diet caused a distortion in crypt structure and total or partial villous atrophy; increased CD4+ T cells, natural killer cells and Qa-1 and NKG2D expression on T cells (two immunomodulatory proteins); and decreased regulatory T cells in intraepithelial lymphocytes. Therefore, TDCA could be used as an early diagnosis biomarker, and more importantly, targeted therapies to eliminate TDCA-producing bacteria (*Clostridium XIVa* and *Clostridium XI*) early in life could be used as a strategy to decrease the CD development risk. On the other hand, they found that the cytokine plasma profile and other metabolites were altered in CD progressors, even before diagnosis (other recent work (Auricchio et al., 2023 [110]) has also focused on the serum cytokine profile and proinflammatory genes expression in infants at CD risk), and differences were also found in the gut microbiota composition (studied in stool) (other authors have also studied microbiota and metabolome alterations in infants at risk of CD, in stool [111,112]). In the CD progressors, before diagnosis, they found significantly increased levels of three proinflammatory cytokines (IFNA2, IL-1a and IL-17E/(IL25)) and a chemokine (MIP-1b/CCl4).

Another interesting aspect to be addressed is alternative biomarkers that allow the disease to be monitored and can also be used in the evaluation of celiac patients' relatives. Plasma citrulline was assessed by an LC auto sampler (and in dried blood spots) by

Lomash et al., 2021 [113], as a potential biomarker useful in the diagnosis and monitoring of the disease, as well as in the evaluation of celiac patients' first-degree relatives (FDRs) (predictive value in the distinction of seronegative CD and in the progression of potential to overt CD). This non-essential amino acid is specifically produced by proximal small intestine enterocyte villi, so it has been proposed as a possible marker of residual intestinal function in pathologies such as necrotizing enterocolitis in newborns, enterophaties, small intestine transplantation or small bowel resections [114]. This work found statistically significant differences in the median plasma citrulline levels in celiac children (20.1 μM (IQR, 13.35–29.15)) compared to controls (serology-negative FDRs) (37.33 μM (IQR, 29.8–42.6)). They also found an inverse correlation between plasma citrulline levels and anti-tTG IgA levels throughout the establishment of GFD and, in addition, in the different Marsh grades at diagnosis; so, citrulline could be used as a surrogate biomarker for serology in disease monitoring and in predicting the histopathological damage degree (it was effective in distinguishing grades 3b and above but not in distinguishing 3a or less in celiac patients and healthy asymptomatic FDRs). In addition, in patients with inconclusive serology and biopsy results, the median plasma citrulline reflected mucosal damage (12.26 μM) like in potential celiacs (median plasma citrulline levels: 23.25 μM). A brief summary of the clinical metabolomic studies conducted on the serum and plasma of children with CD is reviewed in Table 2.

Table 2. Summary of blood metabolomics findings in the selected studies.

Study Reference	Groups (N)	Age	Sample	Methodology	Key Results
[102]	CD progressors (30) vs. HC with similar genetic profiles (20)	0–8 years	Serum	LC-MS, MRM	Altered serum phospholipid profile, even before gluten intake, in CD progressors: Elevated lyso- and PC and PC-O serum levels; Decreased PE 34:1 and PE 36:1 serum levels.
[103]	CD progressors (23) vs. HC matched for HLA risk, sex, and age (23)	0–6 years	Plasma	MS	Altered serum lipid profile in CD progressors: Elevated TGs of low carbon number and double-bond count plasma levels. Decreased PC, cholesterol esters, endogenous TGs and total essential TG plasma levels (these latter after gluten intake).
[105]	CD progressors (33) vs. HC matched for HLA risk (197)	4 month–8 years	Serum	LC-MS/MS	No significant differences; decreased serum phospholipids levels in CD progressors. No influence of HLA genotype on the serum metabolic profile.
[106]	T-CD (17) vs. HC (siblings) (17)	4–17 years	Plasma	LC-MS/MS	Altered plasma lipid profile in T-CD: elevated carboxylic acids and ceramides, diacylglycerides and lysophospholipid plasma levels. Other altered molecules: fatty acyls, glycerolipids, glycerophospholipids, organoxygen compound, sphingolipids, steroid metabolism, molecules involved in bilirubin metabolism.
[108]	T-CD (17) vs. HC (siblings) (17)	4–17 years	Plasma	LC-MS/MS	Altered one-carbon metabolism in T-CD: Trans-sulphuration pathway down-regulation (decreased cysteine and cystathionine plasma levels), with glutathione and vitamin B6 normal levels.

Table 2. *Cont.*

Study Reference	Groups (N)	Age	Sample	Methodology	Key Results
[109]	CD progressors (7 (plasma samples)) vs. HC matched for age, HLA genotype, breastfeeding duration and gluten exposure duration (9 (plasma samples))	2.5–5 years	Plasma, stool	MS, GC-MS, LC-MS, HR-MS	Altered plasma cytokine profile (and other metabolites) in CD progressors: Elevated IFNA2, IL-1a, IL-17E/(IL25)), MIP-1b/CCl4, 2-Methyl-3-ketovalric acid, TDCA, Glucono-D-lactone and Isoburyryl-L-carnitine; Decreased oleic acid plasma levels.
[113]	T-CD (558) vs. HC (FDRs) (1565)	1–18 years (T-CD)	Plasma, DBS	LC-MS, DBS	Decreased plasma citrulline levels in T-CD. Decreased plasma citrulline levels in HLA DQ 2.5-positive patients. Inverse correlation between citrulline levels and anti-tTG IgA levels. Value of citrulline levels as predictors of histopathological damage (Marsh 3b and above).

CD, celiac disease; GFD, gluten-free diet; T-CD, GFD treated celiac disease subjects; HC, healthy controls; CD progressors, children who develop CD; FDRs, first-degree relatives; MS, mass spectrometry; GC-MS, gas chromatography mass spectrometry; LC-MS, liquid chromatography coupled with mass spectrometry; HR-MS, high resolution mass spectrometry; MRM, multiple-reaction monitoring; DBS, dried blood spot; PC, phosphatidylcholines; PC-O, alkylacylphosphatidylcholines; PE, phosphatidylethanolamines; TGs, triacylgycerols; TDCA, taurodeoxycholic acid; HLA, human leukocyte antigen; anti-tTG IgA, anti-tissue transglutaminase IgA.

4.2. Genetic Influence (HLA)

In the above-mentioned work [113], plasma citrulline levels were also correlated with HLA genotype. Significantly low plasma citrulline levels were observed in subjects with the HLA DQ 2.5 genotype with subtypes DQA1*0501 and DQB1*0201. The HLA-DQ genotype has already been reported to influence early intestinal microbial colonization, thus influencing the metabolome [115].

Kirchberg et al. (2016) found that the HLA genotype did not have any influence on the serum metabolic profile in infants who were at risk for celiac disease before introducing gluten to their diet [105].

5. Urine Metabolomic Profile

Other studies (Table 3) have also compared the urine metabolomic profile of celiac children with healthy controls, some of them focusing on changes in the volatile organic compounds (VOCs) profile. An example of this is Di Cagno et al., 2011 [116], who, using gas chromatography mass spectrometry/solid-phase microextraction (GC-MS/SPME) analysis, demonstrated that VOCs and free-amino-acid levels are altered in the urine (and stool) of celiac children with more than 2 years of GFD, relating these imbalances to qualitative and quantitative differences in the microbiota of celiac patients compared to healthy people. They found that the CD group had higher dimethyl trisulfide and dimethyl disulfide urine levels. In addition, with some exceptions, they also had higher urine hydrocarbon levels. No differences in urine aldehyde levels were found between the two groups. These findings were confirmed by NMR, which also found that the CD group had higher lysine, arginine, creatine and methylamine mean levels, while carnosine, glucose, glutamine and 3-methyl-2-oxobutanoic acid were the highest in healthy children. This study emphasizes that a GFD does not completely restore the microbiota or, consequently, the metabolome of children with CD, and that there are possible metabolic markers of CD; furthermore, it suggests that the addition of prebiotics and probiotics to the GFD could restore the microbiota–microbiome balance in celiac children.

Table 3. Summary of urine metabolomics findings in the selected studies.

Study Reference	Groups (N)	Age	Sample	Methodology	Key Results
[116]	T-CD (19) vs. HC (15)	6–12 years	Stool, urine	GC-MS/SPME, H-NMR	Altered VOCs and free-amino-acid levels: - T-CD: elevated dimethyl trisulfide and dimethyl disulfide urine levels and most hydrocarbon levels. Elevated lysine, arginine, creatine and methylamine mean levels: - HC: elevated carnosine, glucose, glutamine and 3-methyl-2-oxobutanoic acid levels.
[117]	T-CD Synergy 1 (11) vs. T-CD placebo (12)	4–18 years	Urine	GC-MS/SPME	No significant changes in VOC urine profiles, except for benzaldehyde concentrations (36% decrease after 12 weeks of intervention).
[118]	T-CD (9) vs. HC (9)	4–14 years	Urine	GC-MS/SPME	Altered VOC levels: - Only in T-CD: 1,3-di-tert-butylbenzene in urine. - HC: elevated 2,3-butanedione, 2-heptanone, dimethyl disulfide and octanal levels (and 2-butanone, hexanal and 4-heptanone).

CD, celiac disease; GFD, gluten-free diet; T-CD, GFD treated celiac disease subjects; HC, healthy controls; GC-MS/SPME, gas chromatography mass spectrometry/solid-phase microextraction; H-NMR, hydrogen-1 nuclear magnetic resonance; VOCs, volatile organic compounds.

In relation to this aspect, Drabinska et al., 2019 [117], studied the effect of GFD supplementation with a prebiotic (oligofructose-enriched inulin) on VOC urine concentration in celiac children and adolescents, using GC-MS/SPME analysis. This work is based on the idea that changes in the VOC profile in biological fluids that occur in various gastrointestinal diseases (studied by the recent so-called "volatolomics") are due in part to alterations in microbiota metabolism, especially its fermentative activity, and not so much to variations in its composition. However, GFD supplementation with this prebiotic had no impact on most VOC urine profiles of celiac patients; only a significant change was observed in benzaldehyde concentrations, which decreased by 36% after 12 weeks of intervention, which may be related to a decrease in *Lactobacillus* counts in the prebiotic-supplemented group, as *Lactobacillus* produces an aminotransferase that converts phenylalanine to benzaldehyde.

Another study, also led by Drabinska [118], aimed to optimize the GC-MS/SPME method for the detection of changes in VOC urine profiles in celiac children compared to healthy children. Based on Variable Importance in the Projection (VIP) scores, several CD biomarkers could be suggested: 1,3-di-tert-butylbenzene (only found in the urine of celiac children) and other VOCs present in higher concentrations in the urine of healthy children (2,3-butanedione, 2-heptanone, dimethyl disulfide and octanal, and, with lower VIP scores, 2-butanone, hexanal and 4-heptanone). Again, these differences could be explained by alterations in the celiac patients' gut microbiota, as many VOCs are fermentation products of the microbiota. On the other hand, the VOC levels in biological fluids (blood, urine, sweat ...) could be increased by the altered intestinal permeability present in many gastrointestinal tract diseases.

6. Discussion

Metabolomics is a promising field that offers a comprehensive understanding of cell biology, surpassing other omics sciences in its breadth. However, the current studies in the field indicate that there is still much progress to be made. The limited number of pediatric studies, often pilot studies, that do not consider the impact of a GFD, contribute to these challenges.

Looking ahead, the potential applications of metabolomics are vast. Diagnostic biomarkers for potential celiacs, the normalization of cellular function alongside the proper implementation of a GFD and the identification of unique disease markers hold promise for deeper insights into CD. Many of the studies mentioned in the literature have primarily focused on analyzing metabolite profiles at a single time point, neglecting the potential influence of the GFD on these profiles. Moreover, there is a lack of consensus regarding the definition of cellular normality in patients. Additionally, it remains inconclusive whether a distinct disease footprint exists, although several studies suggest such a possibility. To address these limitations, it is crucial to design comprehensive studies that encompass metabolomic profiles before disease onset, during the disease with consideration of different treatment approaches and in relation to dietary deviations. Such studies hold the potential to identify valuable biomarkers for effective disease management.

Moreover, to advance our understanding, it is crucial to integrate metabolomic studies with other omics sciences, such as transcriptomics, proteomics and the study of the microbiome. Further studies are needed, as well as studies looking at lipid metabolism and other possible biomarkers. This correlation will help unravel the genetic and epigenetic expressions underlying the observed metabolic findings. Furthermore, the role of the GFD, the importance of well-designed research and the correlation with other omics sciences are key factors for comprehending the disease from a metabolomics perspective.

Most of the studies mentioned have fewer than 30 participants. By fostering increased collaboration among these research groups and facilitating the integration of datasets and participant pools, we can pave the way for large-scale metabolomics research endeavors that possess the required statistical power to establish a definitive diagnostic biomarker for celiac disease. By combining resources and expertise, we can overcome the limitations of individual studies and achieve more robust and conclusive results. This collaborative approach holds tremendous potential for advancing our understanding of celiac disease and improving its diagnosis and management.

Unfortunately, while metabolomics presents exciting possibilities, there is still much to be explored. By refining research methodologies and integrating multiple omics sciences, we can unlock a wealth of information and advance our understanding of CD. Future studies, including larger sample sizes and considering various biological tissues beyond plasma, will provide valuable insights.

7. Conclusions

CD is a multifactorial entity involving genetic and environmental factors. GFD is the only treatment currently available for CD, although solid biomarkers that allow the adequate monitoring of the disease and treatment are still lacking. On the other hand, it would be interesting to find biomarkers that allow the early diagnosis of the disease. In this sense, metabolomics studies may provide answers to the knowledge gaps that exist in CD and other multifactorial disorders, requiring further research in the pediatric age group.

Author Contributions: Conceptualization, R.M.-M. and V.M.N.-L.; methodology, R.M.-M. and M.H.-L.; validation, R.M.-M., R.P. and T.N.; formal analysis, R.M.-M.; investigation, R.M.-M., M.J.-M. and M.H.-L.; resources, R.M.-M., V.M.N.-L. and T.N.; data curation, R.M.-M., M.J.-M. and M.H.-L.; writing—original draft preparation, R.M.-M., M.J.-M., M.H.-L., E.O., M.J., R.P., V.M.N.-L. and T.N.; writing—review and editing, R.M.-M., M.J.-M., M.H.-L., E.O., M.J., R.P., V.M.N.-L. and T.N.; project administration, R.M.-M. and V.M.N.-L.; funding acquisition, R.M.-M. and T.N. All authors have read and agreed to the published version of the manuscript.

Funding: This research was funded by the FEDER/Junta de Andalucía-Consejería de Transformación Económica, Industria, Conocimiento y Universidades Projects FEDER No B-AGR-658 and Excelencia P21_00101. It was also partially funded with the grant "Investigation grant program by the Association of Celiacs and Sensitive to Gluten of the Community of Madrid" and the Government of Catalonia: Agency for the Management of University and Resarch Grants (2021SGR00990). María Jiménez-Muñoz is grateful to the Ph.D. program "Nutrición y Ciencias de los Alimentos" from the University of Granada.

Institutional Review Board Statement: Not applicable.

Informed Consent Statement: Not applicable.

Data Availability Statement: Not applicable.

Acknowledgments: The figure was partly generated using Servier Medical Art, provided by Servier, licensed under a Creative Com-mons Attribution 3.0 unported license.

Conflicts of Interest: The authors declare no conflict of interest.

References

1. Martín-Masot, R.; Diaz-Castro, J.; Moreno-Fernandez, J.; Navas-López, V.M.; Nestares, T. The Role of Early Programming and Early Nutrition on the Development and Progression of Celiac Disease: A Review. *Nutrients* **2020**, *12*, 3427. [CrossRef] [PubMed]
2. Ludvigsson, J.F.; Bai, J.C.; Biagi, F.; Card, T.R.; Ciacci, C.; Ciclitira, P.J.; Green, P.H.R.; Hadjivassiliou, M.; Holdoway, A.; Van Heel, D.A.; et al. Diagnosis and Management of Adult Coeliac Disease: Guidelines from the British Society of Gastroenterology. *Gut* **2014**, *63*, 1210–1228. [CrossRef]
3. Szajewska, H.; Shamir, R.; Mearin, L.; Ribes-Koninckx, C.; Catassi, C.; Domellof, M.; Fewtrell, M.S.; Husby, S.; Papadopoulou, A.; Vandenplas, Y.; et al. Gluten Introduction and the Risk of Coeliac Disease: A Position Paper by the European Society for Pediatric Gastroenterology, Hepatology, and Nutrition. *J. Pediatr. Gastroenterol. Nutr.* **2016**, *62*, 507–513. [CrossRef]
4. Lebwohl, B.; Sanders, D.S.; Green, P.H.R. Coeliac Disease. *Lancet* **2018**, *391*, 70–81. [CrossRef]
5. Caio, G.; Volta, U.; Sapone, A.; Leffler, D.A.; De Giorgio, R.; Catassi, C.; Fasano, A. Celiac Disease: A Comprehensive Current Review. *BMC Med.* **2019**, *17*, 142. [CrossRef]
6. Leonard, M.M.; Karathia, H.; Pujolassos, M.; Troisi, J.; Valitutti, F.; Subramanian, P.; Camhi, S.; Kenyon, V.; Colucci, A.; Serena, G.; et al. Multi-Omics Analysis Reveals the Influence of Genetic and Environmental Risk Factors on Developing Gut Microbiota in Infants at Risk of Celiac Disease. *Microbiome* **2020**, *8*, 130. [CrossRef]
7. King, J.A.; Jeong, J.; Underwood, F.E.; Quan, J.; Panaccione, N.; Windsor, J.W.; Coward, S.; Debruyn, J.; Ronksley, P.E.; Shaheen, A.A.; et al. Incidence of Celiac Disease Is Increasing over Time: A Systematic Review and Meta-Analysis. *Am. J. Gastroenterol.* **2020**, *115*, 507–525. [CrossRef]
8. Abrams, J.A.; Diamond, B.; Rotterdam, H.; Green, P.H.R. Seronegative Celiac Disease: Increased Prevalence with Lesser Degrees of Villous Atrophy. *Dig. Dis. Sci.* **2004**, *49*, 546–550. [CrossRef] [PubMed]
9. Charlesworth, R.P.G. Diagnosing Coeliac Disease: Out with the Old and in with the New? *World J. Gastroenterol.* **2020**, *26*, 1–10. [CrossRef] [PubMed]
10. Simpson, S.M.; Ciaccio, E.J.; Case, S.; Jaffe, N.; Mahadov, S.; Lebwohl, B.; Green, P.H. Celiac Disease in Patients with Type 1 Diabetes: Screening and Diagnostic Practices. *Diabetes Educ.* **2013**, *39*, 532–540. [CrossRef]
11. Volta, U.; Rostami, K.; Tovoli, F.; Caio, G.; Masi, C.; Ruggeri, E.; Cacciari, G.; Bon, I.; De Giorgio, R. Fulminant Type 1 Autoimmune Hepatitis in a Recently Diagnosed Celiac Disease Patient. *Arch. Iran Med.* **2013**, *16*, 683–685. [PubMed]
12. Martín-Masot, R.; Herrador-López, M.; Navas-López, V.M.; Carmona, F.D.; Nestares, T.; Bossini-Castillo, L. Celiac Disease Is a Risk Factor for Mature T and NK Cell Lymphoma: A Mendelian Randomization Study. *Int. J. Mol. Sci.* **2023**, *24*, 7216. [CrossRef]
13. Diaz-Castro, J.; Muriel-Neyra, C.; Martin-Masot, R.; Moreno-Fernandez, J.; Maldonado, J.; Nestares, T. Oxidative Stress, DNA Stability and Evoked Inflammatory Signaling in Young Celiac Patients Consuming a Gluten-Free Diet. *Eur. J. Nutr.* **2019**, *59*, 1577–1584. [CrossRef] [PubMed]
14. Nestares, T.; Martín-Masot, R.; Flor-Alemany, M.; Bonavita, A.; Maldonado, J.; Aparicio, V.A. Influence of Ultra-Processed Foods Consumption on Redox Status and Inflammatory Signaling in Young Celiac Patients. *Nutrients* **2021**, *13*, 156. [CrossRef] [PubMed]
15. Nestares, T.; Martín-Masot, R.; Labella, A.; Aparicio, V.A.; Flor-Alemany, M.; López-Frías, M.; Maldonado, J. Is a Gluten-Free Diet Enough to Maintain Correct Micronutrients Status in Young Patients with Celiac Disease? *Nutrients* **2020**, *12*, 844. [CrossRef]
16. Silano, M.; Volta, U.; Mecchia, A.M.; Dessì, M.; Di Benedetto, R.; De Vincenzi, M. Delayed Diagnosis of Coeliac Disease Increases Cancer Risk. *BMC Gastroenterol.* **2007**, *7*, 8. [CrossRef]
17. Viljamaa, M.; Kaukinen, K.; Pukkala, E.; Hervonen, K.; Reunala, T.; Collin, P. Malignancies and Mortality in Patients with Coeliac Disease and Dermatitis Herpetiformis: 30-Year Population-Based Study. *Dig. Liver Dis.* **2006**, *38*, 374–380. [CrossRef]
18. Mearin, M.L.; Catassi, C.; Brousse, N.; Brand, R.; Collin, P.; Fabiani, E.; Schweizer, J.J.; Abuzakouk, M.; Szajewska, H.; Hallert, C.; et al. European Multi-Centre Study on Coeliac Disease and Non-Hodgkin Lymphoma. *Eur. J. Gastroenterol. Hepatol.* **2006**, *18*, 187–194. [CrossRef]
19. Ilus, T.; Kaukinen, K.; Virta, L.J.; Pukkala, E.; Collin, P. Incidence of Malignancies in Diagnosed Celiac Patients: A Population-Based Estimate. *Am. J. Gastroenterol.* **2014**, *109*, 1471–1477. [CrossRef]
20. Kell, D.B.; Goodacre, R. Metabolomics and Systems Pharmacology: Why and How to Model the Human Metabolic Network for Drug Discovery. *Drug Discov. Today* **2014**, *19*, 171–182. [CrossRef]
21. Allen, J.; Davey, H.M.; Broadhurst, D.; Heald, J.K.; Rowland, J.J.; Oliver, S.G.; Kell, D.B. High-Throughput Classification of Yeast Mutants for Functional Genomics Using Metabolic Footprinting. *Nat. Biotechnol.* **2003**, *21*, 692–696. [CrossRef]

22. Sellitto, M.; Bai, G.; Serena, G.; Fricke, W.F.; Sturgeon, C.; Gajer, P.; White, J.R.; Koenig, S.S.K.; Sakamoto, J.; Boothe, D.; et al. Proof of Concept of Microbiome-Metabolome Analysis and Delayed Gluten Exposure on Celiac Disease Autoimmunity in Genetically at-Risk Infants. *PLoS ONE* **2012**, *7*, e33387. [CrossRef]
23. Nicholson, J.K.; Lindon, J.C.; Holmes, E. "Metabonomics": Understanding the Metabolic Responses of Living Systems to Pathophysiological Stimuli via Multivariate Statistical Analysis of Biological NMR Spectroscopic Data. *Xenobiotica* **1999**, *29*, 1181–1189. [CrossRef] [PubMed]
24. Evans, A.M.; DeHaven, C.D.; Barrett, T.; Mitchell, M.; Milgram, E. Integrated, Nontargeted Ultrahigh Performance Liquid Chromatography/Electrospray Ionization Tandem Mass Spectrometry Platform for the Identification and Relative Quantification of the Small-Molecule Complement of Biological Systems. *Anal. Chem.* **2009**, *81*, 6656–6667. [CrossRef] [PubMed]
25. Dunn, W.B. Current Trends and Future Requirements for the Mass Spectrometric Investigation of Microbial, Mammalian and Plant Metabolomes. *Phys. Biol.* **2008**, *5*, 011001. [CrossRef] [PubMed]
26. Kan, M.; Himes, B.E. Insights into Glucocorticoid Responses Derived from Omics Studies. *Pharmacol. Ther.* **2021**, *218*, 107674. [CrossRef] [PubMed]
27. Bordag, N.; Klie, S.; Jürchott, K.; Vierheller, J.; Schiewe, H.; Albrecht, V.; Tonn, J.-C.; Schwartz, C.; Schichor, C.; Selbig, J. Glucocorticoid (Dexamethasone)-Induced Metabolome Changes in Healthy Males Suggest Prediction of Response and Side Effects. *Sci. Rep.* **2015**, *5*, 15954. [CrossRef] [PubMed]
28. Wishart, D.S. Emerging Applications of Metabolomics in Drug Discovery and Precision Medicine. *Nat. Rev. Drug Discov.* **2016**, *15*, 473–484. [CrossRef]
29. Johnson, C.H.; Ivanisevic, J.; Siuzdak, G. Metabolomics: Beyond Biomarkers and towards Mechanisms. *Nat. Rev. Mol. Cell Biol.* **2016**, *17*, 451–459. [CrossRef]
30. Petrick, L.; Edmands, W.; Schiffman, C.; Grigoryan, H.; Perttula, K.; Yano, Y.; Dudoit, S.; Whitehead, T.; Metayer, C.; Rappaport, S. An Untargeted Metabolomics Method for Archived Newborn Dried Blood Spots in Epidemiologic Studies. *Metabolomics* **2017**, *13*, 27. [CrossRef]
31. Niedzwiecki, M.M.; Walker, D.I.; Vermeulen, R.; Chadeau-Hyam, M.; Jones, D.P.; Miller, G.W. The Exposome: Molecules to Populations. *Annu. Rev. Pharmacol. Toxicol.* **2019**, *59*, 107–127. [CrossRef] [PubMed]
32. Johnson, J.M.; Yu, T.; Strobel, F.H.; Jones, D.P. A Practical Approach to Detect Unique Metabolic Patterns for Personalized Medicine. *Analyst* **2010**, *135*, 2864. [CrossRef] [PubMed]
33. Cabré, R.; Jové, M.; Naudí, A.; Ayala, V.; Piñol-Ripoll, G.; Gil-Villar, M.P.; Dominguez-Gonzalez, M.; Obis, È.; Berdun, R.; Mota-Martorell, N.; et al. Specific Metabolomics Adaptations Define a Differential Regional Vulnerability in the Adult Human Cerebral Cortex. *Front. Mol. Neurosci.* **2016**, *9*, 138. [CrossRef]
34. Goodpaster, B.H.; Sparks, L.M. Metabolic Flexibility in Health and Disease. *Cell Metab.* **2017**, *25*, 1027–1036. [CrossRef]
35. Moreau, R.; Clària, J.; Aguilar, F.; Fenaille, F.; Lozano, J.J.; Junot, C.; Colsch, B.; Caraceni, P.; Trebicka, J.; Pavesi, M.; et al. Blood Metabolomics Uncovers Inflammation-Associated Mitochondrial Dysfunction as a Potential Mechanism Underlying ACLF. *J. Hepatol.* **2020**, *72*, 688–701. [CrossRef]
36. Pang, H.; Jia, W.; Hu, Z. Emerging Applications of Metabolomics in Clinical Pharmacology. *Clin. Pharmacol. Ther.* **2019**, *106*, 544–556. [CrossRef] [PubMed]
37. Zhang, A.; Sun, H.; Wang, X. Power of Metabolomics in Biomarker Discovery and Mining Mechanisms of Obesity. *Obes. Rev.* **2013**, *14*, 344–349. [CrossRef]
38. Thomson, T.M.; Balcells, C.; Cascante, M. Metabolic Plasticity and Epithelial-Mesenchymal Transition. *J. Clin. Med.* **2019**, *8*, 967. [CrossRef] [PubMed]
39. Saner, C.; Harcourt, B.E.; Pandey, A.; Ellul, S.; McCallum, Z.; Kao, K.-T.; Twindyakirana, C.; Pons, A.; Alexander, E.J.; Saffery, R.; et al. Sex and Puberty-Related Differences in Metabolomic Profiles Associated with Adiposity Measures in Youth with Obesity. *Metabolomics* **2019**, *15*, 75. [CrossRef] [PubMed]
40. Handelman, S.K.; Romero, R.; Tarca, A.L.; Pacora, P.; Ingram, B.; Maymon, E.; Chaiworapongsa, T.; Hassan, S.S.; Erez, O. The Plasma Metabolome of Women in Early Pregnancy Differs from That of Non-Pregnant Women. *PLoS ONE* **2019**, *14*, e224682. [CrossRef] [PubMed]
41. Christian, P.; Smith, E.R.; Lee, S.E.; Vargas, A.J.; Bremer, A.A.; Raiten, D.J. The Need to Study Human Milk as a Biological System. *Am. J. Clin. Nutr.* **2021**, *113*, 1063–1072. [CrossRef] [PubMed]
42. Mota-Martorell, N.; Jové, M.; Borrás, C.; Berdún, R.; Obis, È.; Sol, J.; Cabré, R.; Pradas, I.; Galo-Licona, J.D.; Puig, J.; et al. Methionine Transsulfuration Pathway Is Upregulated in Long-Lived Humans. *Free Radic. Biol. Med.* **2021**, *162*, 38–52. [CrossRef] [PubMed]
43. Sol, J.; Obis, È.; Mota-Martorell, N.; Pradas, I.; Galo-Licona, J.D.; Martin-Garí, M.; Fernández-Bernal, A.; Ortega-Bravo, M.; Mayneris-Perxachs, J.; Borrás, C.; et al. Plasma Acylcarnitines and Gut-derived Aromatic Amino Acids as Sex-specific Hub Metabolites of the Human Aging Metabolome. *Aging Cell* **2023**, *22*, e13821. [CrossRef] [PubMed]
44. Sas, K.M.; Karnovsky, A.; Michailidis, G.; Pennathur, S. Metabolomics and Diabetes: Analytical and Computational Approaches. *Diabetes* **2015**, *64*, 718–732. [CrossRef] [PubMed]
45. Wang-Sattler, R.; Yu, Z.; Herder, C.; Messias, A.C.; Floegel, A.; He, Y.; Heim, K.; Campillos, M.; Holzapfel, C.; Thorand, B.; et al. Novel Biomarkers for Pre-diabetes Identified by Metabolomics. *Mol. Syst. Biol.* **2012**, *8*, 615. [CrossRef]

46. Pallares-Méndez, R.; Aguilar-Salinas, C.A.; Cruz-Bautista, I.; del Bosque-Plata, L. Metabolomics in Diabetes, a Review. *Ann. Med.* **2016**, *48*, 89–102. [CrossRef]
47. Danzi, F.; Pacchiana, R.; Mafficini, A.; Scupoli, M.T.; Scarpa, A.; Donadelli, M.; Fiore, A. To Metabolomics and beyond: A Technological Portfolio to Investigate Cancer Metabolism. *Signal Transduct. Target Ther.* **2023**, *8*, 137. [CrossRef]
48. Gatius, S.; Jove, M.; Megino-Luque, C.; Albertí-Valls, M.; Yeramian, A.; Bonifaci, N.; Piñol, M.; Santacana, M.; Pradas, I.; Llobet-Navas, D.; et al. Metabolomic Analysis Points to Bioactive Lipid Species and Acireductone Dioxygenase 1 (ADI1) as Potential Therapeutic Targets in Poor Prognosis Endometrial Cancer. *Cancers* **2022**, *14*, 2842. [CrossRef]
49. Shao, Y.; Le, W. Recent Advances and Perspectives of Metabolomics-Based Investigations in Parkinson's Disease. *Mol. Neurodegener.* **2019**, *14*, 3. [CrossRef]
50. Pamplona, R.; Obis, E.; Sol, J.; Andres-Benito, P.; Martí n-Gari, M.; Mota-Martorell, N.; Daniel Galo-Licona, J.; Piñol-Ripoll, G.; Portero-Otin, M.; Ferrer, I.; et al. Lipidomic Alterations in the Cerebral Cortex and White Matter in Sporadic Alzheimer's Disease. *bioRxiv* **2023**. [CrossRef]
51. Centanni, M.; Moes, D.J.A.R.; Trocóniz, I.F.; Ciccolini, J.; van Hasselt, J.G.C. Clinical Pharmacokinetics and Pharmacodynamics of Immune Checkpoint Inhibitors. *Clin. Pharmacokinet.* **2019**, *58*, 835–857. [CrossRef]
52. Alarcon-Barrera, J.C.; Kostidis, S.; Ondo-Mendez, A.; Giera, M. Recent Advances in Metabolomics Analysis for Early Drug Development. *Drug Discov. Today* **2022**, *27*, 1763–1773. [CrossRef]
53. De Castro, F.; Benedetti, M.; Del Coco, L.; Fanizzi, F.P. NMR-Based Metabolomics in Metal-Based Drug Research. *Molecules* **2019**, *24*, 2240. [CrossRef]
54. Lindon, J.C.; Holmes, E.; Nicholson, J.K. Metabonomics in Pharmaceutical R & D. *FEBS J.* **2007**, *274*, 1140–1151.
55. Uppal, K.; Walker, D.I.; Liu, K.; Li, S.; Go, Y.-M.; Jones, D.P. Computational Metabolomics: A Framework for the Million Metabolome. *Chem. Res. Toxicol.* **2016**, *29*, 1956–1975. [CrossRef] [PubMed]
56. Yoon, D.; Lee, M.; Kim, S.; Kim, S. Applications of NMR Spectroscopy Based Metabolomics: A Review. *J. Korean Magn. Reson. Soc.* **2013**, *17*, 1–10. [CrossRef]
57. Kim, J.U.; Shariff, M.I.F.; Crossey, M.M.E.; Gomez-Romero, M.; Holmes, E.; Cox, I.J.; Fye, H.K.S.; Njie, R.; Taylor-Robinson, S.D. Hepatocellular Carcinoma: Review of Disease and Tumor Biomarkers. *World J. Hepatol.* **2016**, *8*, 471. [CrossRef]
58. Emwas, A.-H.M. The Strengths and Weaknesses of NMR Spectroscopy and Mass Spectrometry with Particular Focus on Metabolomics Research. In *Metabonomics: Methods and Protocols*; Springer: Berlin/Heidelberg, Germany, 2015; pp. 161–193.
59. Adamski, J. Introduction to Metabolomics. In *Metabolomics for Biomedical Research*; Elsevier: Amsterdam, The Netherlands, 2020; pp. 1–15.
60. Bhinderwala, F.; Wase, N.; DiRusso, C.; Powers, R. Combining Mass Spectrometry and NMR Improves Metabolite Detection and Annotation. *J. Proteome Res.* **2018**, *17*, 4017–4022. [CrossRef] [PubMed]
61. Emwas, A.-H.; Roy, R.; McKay, R.T.; Tenori, L.; Saccenti, E.; Gowda, G.A.N.; Raftery, D.; Alahmari, F.; Jaremko, L.; Jaremko, M.; et al. NMR Spectroscopy for Metabolomics Research. *Metabolites* **2019**, *9*, 123. [CrossRef]
62. Keun, H.C.; Athersuch, T.J. Nuclear Magnetic Resonance (NMR)-Based Metabolomics. In *Metabolic Profiling: Methods and Protocols*; Springer: Berlin/Heidelberg, Germany, 2011; pp. 321–334.
63. Letertre, M.P.M.; Dervilly, G.; Giraudeau, P. Combined Nuclear Magnetic Resonance Spectroscopy and Mass Spectrometry Approaches for Metabolomics. *Anal. Chem.* **2021**, *93*, 500–518. [CrossRef] [PubMed]
64. Psychogios, N.; Hau, D.D.; Peng, J.; Guo, A.C.; Mandal, R.; Bouatra, S.; Sinelnikov, I.; Krishnamurthy, R.; Eisner, R.; Gautam, B.; et al. The Human Serum Metabolome. *PLoS ONE* **2011**, *6*, e16957. [CrossRef]
65. Junot, C.; Fenaille, F.; Colsch, B.; Bécher, F. High Resolution Mass Spectrometry Based Techniques at the Crossroads of Metabolic Pathways. *Mass Spectrom. Rev.* **2014**, *33*, 471–500. [CrossRef] [PubMed]
66. Yanes, O.; Tautenhahn, R.; Patti, G.J.; Siuzdak, G. Expanding Coverage of the Metabolome for Global Metabolite Profiling. *Anal. Chem.* **2011**, *83*, 2152–2161. [CrossRef] [PubMed]
67. Piraud, M.; Vianey-Saban, C.; Petritis, K.; Elfakir, C.; Steghens, J.; Morla, A.; Bouchu, D. ESI-MS/MS Analysis of Underivatised Amino Acids: A New Tool for the Diagnosis of Inherited Disorders of Amino Acid Metabolism. Fragmentation Study of 79 Molecules of Biological Interest in Positive and Negative Ionisation Mode. *Rapid Commun. Mass Spectrom.* **2003**, *17*, 1297–1311. [CrossRef]
68. Bruins, A.P. Mass spectrometry—Atmospheric Pressure Ionization Techniques. In *Encyclopedia of Analytical Science*; Elsevier: Amsterdam, The Netherlands, 2005; pp. 366–373.
69. Schuhmacher, J.; Zimmer, D.; Tesche, F.; Pickard, V. Matrix Effects during Analysis of Plasma Samples by Electrospray and Atmospheric Pressure Chemical Ionization Mass Spectrometry: Practical Approaches to Their Elimination. *Rapid Commun. Mass Spectrom.* **2003**, *17*, 1950–1957. [CrossRef]
70. Karas, M.; Krüger, R. Ion Formation in MALDI: The Cluster Ionization Mechanism. *Chem. Rev.* **2003**, *103*, 427–440. [CrossRef]
71. Theodoridis, G.; Gika, H.G.; Wilson, I.D. Mass Spectrometry-Based Holistic Analytical Approaches for Metabolite Profiling in Systems Biology Studies. *Mass Spectrom. Rev.* **2011**, *30*, 884–906. [CrossRef]
72. Want, E.J.; Masson, P.; Michopoulos, F.; Wilson, I.D.; Theodoridis, G.; Plumb, R.S.; Shockcor, J.; Loftus, N.; Holmes, E.; Nicholson, J.K. Global Metabolic Profiling of Animal and Human Tissues via UPLC-MS. *Nat. Protoc.* **2013**, *8*, 17–32. [CrossRef] [PubMed]
73. Špánik, I.; Machyňáková, A. Recent Applications of Gas Chromatography with High-Resolution Mass Spectrometry. *J. Sep. Sci.* **2018**, *41*, 163–179. [CrossRef] [PubMed]

74. Zeki, Ö.C.; Eylem, C.C.; Reçber, T.; Kır, S.; Nemutlu, E. Integration of GC–MS and LC–MS for Untargeted Metabolomics Profiling. *J. Pharm. Biomed. Anal.* **2020**, *190*, 113509. [CrossRef] [PubMed]
75. Marshall, D.D.; Powers, R. Beyond the Paradigm: Combining Mass Spectrometry and Nuclear Magnetic Resonance for Metabolomics. *Prog. Nucl. Magn. Reason. Spectrosc.* **2017**, *100*, 1–16. [CrossRef] [PubMed]
76. Martias, C.; Baroukh, N.; Mavel, S.; Blasco, H.; Lefèvre, A.; Roch, L.; Montigny, F.; Gatien, J.; Schibler, L.; Dufour-Rainfray, D.; et al. Optimization of Sample Preparation for Metabolomics Exploration of Urine, Feces, Blood and Saliva in Humans Using Combined NMR and UHPLC-HRMS Platforms. *Molecules* **2021**, *26*, 4111. [CrossRef] [PubMed]
77. Vuckovic, D. Sample Preparation in Global Metabolomics of Biological Fluids and Tissues. In *Proteomic and Metabolomic Approaches to Biomarker Discovery*; Elsevier: Amsterdam, The Netherlands, 2013; pp. 51–75.
78. Lu, W.; Bennett, B.D.; Rabinowitz, J.D. Analytical Strategies for LC–MS-Based Targeted Metabolomics. *J. Chromatogr. B* **2008**, *871*, 236–242. [CrossRef]
79. Patti, G.J.; Tautenhahn, R.; Siuzdak, G. Meta-Analysis of Untargeted Metabolomic Data from Multiple Profiling Experiments. *Nat. Protoc.* **2012**, *7*, 508–516. [CrossRef]
80. Jacob, M.; Malkawi, A.; Albast, N.; Al Bougha, S.; Lopata, A.; Dasouki, M.; Abdel Rahman, A.M. A Targeted Metabolomics Approach for Clinical Diagnosis of Inborn Errors of Metabolism. *Anal. Chim. Acta* **2018**, *1025*, 141–153. [CrossRef] [PubMed]
81. Puigarnau, S.; Fernàndez, A.; Obis, E.; Jové, M.; Castañer, M.; Pamplona, R.; Portero-Otin, M.; Camerino, O. Metabolomics Reveals That Fittest Trail Runners Show a Better Adaptation of Bioenergetic Pathways. *J. Sci. Med. Sport* **2022**, *25*, 6. [CrossRef] [PubMed]
82. Dunn, W.B.; Broadhurst, D.; Begley, P.; Zelena, E.; Francis-McIntyre, S.; Anderson, N.; Brown, M.; Knowles, J.D.; Halsall, A.; Haselden, J.N.; et al. Procedures for Large-Scale Metabolic Profiling of Serum and Plasma Using Gas Chromatography and Liquid Chromatography Coupled to Mass Spectrometry. *Nat. Protoc.* **2011**, *6*, 1060–1083. [CrossRef]
83. Molnos, S.; Wahl, S.; Haid, M.; Eekhoff, E.M.W.; Pool, R.; Floegel, A.; Deelen, J.; Much, D.; Prehn, C.; Breier, M.; et al. Metabolite Ratios as Potential Biomarkers for Type 2 Diabetes: A DIRECT Study. *Diabetologia* **2018**, *61*, 117–129. [CrossRef]
84. Newgard, C.B. Metabolomics and Metabolic Diseases: Where Do We Stand? *Cell Metab.* **2017**, *25*, 43–56. [CrossRef]
85. Phapale, P. Pharmaco-metabolomics Opportunities in Drug Development and Clinical Research. *Anal. Sci. Adv.* **2021**, *2*, 611–616. [CrossRef]
86. Zhang, M.; Yang, H. Perspectives from Metabolomics in the Early Diagnosis and Prognosis of Gestational Diabetes Mellitus. *Front. Endocrinol.* **2022**, *13*, 7191. [CrossRef] [PubMed]
87. Mickiewicz, B.; Vogel, H.J.; Wong, H.R.; Winston, B.W. Metabolomics as a Novel Approach for Early Diagnosis of Pediatric Septic Shock and Its Mortality. *Am. J. Respir Crit. Care Med.* **2013**, *187*, 967–976. [CrossRef]
88. Kaddurah-Daouk, R.; Krishnan, K.R.R. Metabolomics: A Global Biochemical Approach to the Study of Central Nervous System Diseases. *Neuropsychopharmacology* **2009**, *34*, 173–186. [CrossRef]
89. Mock, A.; Zschäbitz, S.; Kirsten, R.; Scheffler, M.; Wolf, B.; Herold-Mende, C.; Kramer, R.; Busch, E.; Jenzer, M.; Jäger, D.; et al. Serum Very Long-Chain Fatty Acid-Containing Lipids Predict Response to Immune Checkpoint Inhibitors in Urological Cancers. *Cancer Immunol. Immunother.* **2019**, *68*, 2005–2014. [CrossRef] [PubMed]
90. Paglia, G.; Williams, J.P.; Menikarachchi, L.; Thompson, J.W.; Tyldesley-Worster, R.; Halldórsson, S.; Rolfsson, O.; Moseley, A.; Grant, D.; Langridge, J.; et al. Ion Mobility Derived Collision Cross Sections to Support Metabolomics Applications. *Anal. Chem.* **2014**, *86*, 3985–3993. [CrossRef] [PubMed]
91. Paglia, G.; Kliman, M.; Claude, E.; Geromanos, S.; Astarita, G. Applications of Ion-Mobility Mass Spectrometry for Lipid Analysis. *Anal. Bioanal. Chem.* **2015**, *407*, 4995–5007. [CrossRef] [PubMed]
92. Paglia, G.; Smith, A.J.; Astarita, G. Ion Mobility Mass Spectrometry in the Omics Era: Challenges and Opportunities for Metabolomics and Lipidomics. *Mass Spectrom. Rev.* **2022**, *41*, 722–765. [CrossRef]
93. Heuillet, M.; Bellvert, F.; Cahoreau, E.; Letisse, F.; Millard, P.; Portais, J.-C. Methodology for the Validation of Isotopic Analyses by Mass Spectrometry in Stable-Isotope Labeling Experiments. *Anal. Chem.* **2018**, *90*, 1852–1860. [CrossRef]
94. Winter, G.; Krömer, J.O. Fluxomics—Connecting 'omics Analysis and Phenotypes. *Environ. Microbiol.* **2013**, *15*, 1901–1916. [CrossRef]
95. Emwas, A.-H.; Szczepski, K.; Al-Younis, I.; Lachowicz, J.I.; Jaremko, M. Fluxomics—New Metabolomics Approaches to Monitor Metabolic Pathways. *Front. Pharmacol.* **2022**, *13*, 5782. [CrossRef]
96. Jang, C.; Chen, L.; Rabinowitz, J.D. Metabolomics and Isotope Tracing. *Cell* **2018**, *173*, 822–837. [CrossRef]
97. Eggers, L.F.; Schwudke, D. Shotgun Lipidomics Approach for Clinical Samples. *Methods Mol. Biol.* **2018**, *1730*, 163–174. [CrossRef]
98. Chekmeneva, E.; dos Santos Correia, G.; Chan, Q.; Wijeyesekera, A.; Tin, A.; Young, J.H.; Elliott, P.; Nicholson, J.K.; Holmes, E. Optimization and Application of Direct Infusion Nanoelectrospray HRMS Method for Large-Scale Urinary Metabolic Phenotyping in Molecular Epidemiology. *J. Proteom. Res.* **2017**, *16*, 1646–1658. [CrossRef]
99. Taylor, M.J.; Lukowski, J.K.; Anderton, C.R. Spatially Resolved Mass Spectrometry at the Single Cell: Recent Innovations in Proteomics and Metabolomics. *J. Am. Soc. Mass Spectrom.* **2021**, *32*, 872–894. [CrossRef] [PubMed]
100. Miura, D.; Fujimura, Y.; Wariishi, H. In Situ Metabolomic Mass Spectrometry Imaging: Recent Advances and Difficulties. *J. Proteom.* **2012**, *75*, 5052–5060. [CrossRef]

101. Abu Sammour, D.; Cairns, J.L.; Boskamp, T.; Marsching, C.; Kessler, T.; Ramallo Guevara, C.; Panitz, V.; Sadik, A.; Cordes, J.; Schmidt, S.; et al. Spatial Probabilistic Mapping of Metabolite Ensembles in Mass Spectrometry Imaging. *Nat. Commun.* **2023**, *14*, 1823. [CrossRef] [PubMed]
102. Auricchio, R.; Galatola, M.; Cielo, D.; Amoresano, A.; Caterino, M.; De Vita, E.; Illiano, A.; Troncone, R.; Greco, L.; Ruoppolo, M. A Phospholipid Profile at 4 Months Predicts the Onset of Celiac Disease in At-Risk Infants. *Sci. Rep.* **2019**, *9*, 14303. [CrossRef] [PubMed]
103. Sen, P.; Carlsson, C.; Virtanen, S.M.; Simell, S.; Hyöty, H.; Ilonen, J.; Toppari, J.; Veijola, R.; Hyötyläinen, T.; Knip, M.; et al. Persistent Alterations in Plasma Lipid Profiles Before Introduction of Gluten in the Diet Associated with Progression to Celiac Disease. *Clin. Transl. Gastroenterol.* **2019**, *10*, 44. [CrossRef]
104. Orešič, M.; Hyötyläinen, T.; Kotronen, A.; Gopalacharyulu, P.; Nygren, H.; Arola, J.; Castillo, S.; Mattila, I.; Hakkarainen, A.; Borra, R.J.H.; et al. Prediction of Non-Alcoholic Fatty-Liver Disease and Liver Fat Content by Serum Molecular Lipids. *Diabetologia* **2013**, *56*, 2266–2274. [CrossRef]
105. Kirchberg, F.F.; Werkstetter, K.J.; Uhl, O.; Auricchio, R.; Castillejo, G.; Korponay-Szabo, I.R.; Polanco, I.; Ribes-Koninckx, C.; Vriezinga, S.L.; Koletzko, B.; et al. Investigating the Early Metabolic Fingerprint of Celiac Disease—A Prospective Approach. *J. Autoimmun.* **2016**, *72*, 95–101. [CrossRef]
106. Martín-Masot, R.; Galo-Licona, J.D.; Mota-Martorell, N.; Sol, J.; Jové, M.; Maldonado, J.; Pamplona, R.; Nestares, T. Up-Regulation of Specific Bioactive Lipids in Celiac Disease. *Nutrients* **2021**, *13*, 2271. [CrossRef] [PubMed]
107. Sedda, S.; Dinallo, V.; Marafini, I.; Franzè, E.; Paoluzi, O.A.; Izzo, R.; Giuffrida, P.; Di Sabatino, A.; Corazza, G.R.; Monteleone, G. MTOR Sustains Inflammatory Response in Celiac Disease. *Sci. Rep.* **2020**, *10*, 10798. [CrossRef]
108. Martín-Masot, R.; Mota-Martorell, N.; Jové, M.; Maldonado, J.; Pamplona, R.; Nestares, T. Alterations in One-Carbon Metabolism in Celiac Disease. *Nutrients* **2020**, *12*, 3723. [CrossRef] [PubMed]
109. Girdhar, K.; Dogru, Y.D.; Huang, Q.; Yang, Y.; Tolstikov, V.; Raisingani, A.; Chrudinova, M.; Oh, J.; Kelley, K.; Ludvigsson, J.F.; et al. Dynamics of the Gut Microbiome, IgA Response, and Plasma Metabolome in the Development of Pediatric Celiac Disease. *Microbiome* **2023**, *11*, 9. [CrossRef]
110. Auricchio, R.; Galatola, M.; Cielo, D.; Rotondo, R.; Carbone, F.; Mandile, R.; Carpinelli, M.; Vitale, S.; Matarese, G.; Gianfrani, C.; et al. Antibody Profile, Gene Expression and Serum Cytokines in At-Risk Infants before the Onset of Celiac Disease. *Int. J. Mol. Sci.* **2023**, *24*, 6836. [CrossRef] [PubMed]
111. Fasano, A.; Leonard, M.M.; Kenyon, V.; Valitutti, F.; Pennacchio-Harrington, R.; Piemontese, P.; Francavilla, R.; Norsa, L.; Passaro, T.; Crocco, M.; et al. Cohort Profile: Celiac Disease Genomic, Environmental, Microbiome and Metabolome Study; a Prospective Longitudinal Birth Cohort Study of Children at-Risk for Celiac Disease. *PLoS ONE* **2023**, *18*, e2082739. [CrossRef]
112. Leonard, M.M.; Valitutti, F.; Karathia, H.; Pujolassos, M.; Kenyon, V.; Fanelli, B.; Troisi, J.; Subramanian, P.; Camhi, S.; Colucci, A.; et al. Microbiome Signatures of Progression toward Celiac Disease Onset in At-Risk Children in a Longitudinal Prospective Cohort Study. *Proc. Natl. Acad. Sci. USA* **2021**, *118*, e2020322118. [CrossRef]
113. Lomash, A.; Prasad, A.; Singh, R.; Kumar, S.; Gupta, R.; Dholakia, D.; Kumar, P.; Batra, V.V.; Puri, A.S.; Kapoor, S. Evaluation of the Utility of Amino Acid Citrulline as a Surrogate Metabolomic Biomarker for the Diagnosis of Celiac Disease. *Nutr. Metab. Insights* **2021**, *14*, 603. [CrossRef]
114. Crenn, P.; Messing, B.; Cynober, L. Citrulline as a Biomarker of Intestinal Failure Due to Enterocyte Mass Reduction. *Clin. Nutr.* **2008**, *27*, 328–339. [CrossRef]
115. Olivares, M.; Albrecht, S.; De Palma, G.; Ferrer, M.D.; Castillejo, G.; Schols, H.A.; Sanz, Y. Human Milk Composition Differs in Healthy Mothers and Mothers with Celiac Disease. *Eur. J. Nutr.* **2015**, *54*, 119–128. [CrossRef]
116. Di Cagno, R.; De Angelis, M.; De Pasquale, I.; Ndagijimana, M.; Vernocchi, P.; Ricciuti, P.; Gagliardi, F.; Laghi, L.; Crecchio, C.; Guerzoni, M.; et al. Duodenal and Faecal Microbiota of Celiac Children: Molecular, Phenotype and Metabolome Characterization. *BMC Microbiol.* **2011**, *11*, 219. [CrossRef] [PubMed]
117. Drabinska, N.; Jarocka-Cyrta, E.; Ratcliffe, N.M.; Krupa-Kozak, U. The Profile of Urinary Headspace Volatile Organic Compounds After 12-Week Intake of Oligofructose-Enriched Inulin by Children and Adolescents with Celiac Disease on a Gluten-Free Diet: Results of a Pilot, Randomized, Placebo-Controlled Clinical Trial. *Molecules* **2019**, *24*, 1341. [CrossRef] [PubMed]
118. Drabińska, N.; Azeem, H.A.; Krupa-Kozak, U. A Targeted Metabolomic Protocol for Quantitative Analysis of Volatile Organic Compounds in Urine of Children with Celiac Disease. *RSC Adv.* **2018**, *8*, 36534–36541. [CrossRef] [PubMed]

nutrients

MDPI

Review

Fertility in Celiac Disease: The Impact of Gluten on Male and Female Reproductive Health

Herbert Wieser [1], Carolina Ciacci [2,*], Carlo Soldaini [2], Carolina Gizzi [2], Lucienne Pellegrini [2] and Antonella Santonicola [2]

[1] Hamburg School of Food Science, Institute of Food Chemistry, University of Hamburg, 20146 Hamburg, Germany; h.wieser2@gmx.de
[2] Gastrointestinal Unit, Department of Medicine, Surgery and Dentistry "Scuola Medica Salernitana", University of Salerno, 84131 Salerno, Italy; carlo.soldaini@outlook.com (C.S.); carolinagizzi@libero.it (C.G.); lucienne.pellegrini@sangiovannieruggi.it (L.P.); asantonicola@unisa.it (A.S.)
* Correspondence: cciacci@unisa.it

Abstract: Celiac disease (CeD) is a chronic immune-mediated disorder of the small intestine triggered by the ingestion of dietary gluten. This narrative review aims to summarize and critically evaluate the recent literature on the association between CeD and infertility, with an emphasis on identifying patterns and inconsistencies. Previous studies have reported conflicting findings: while some demonstrate a higher prevalence of unexplained infertility in patients with CeD, others do not support this association. Overall, untreated CeD may be a contributing factor to infertility, especially unexplained cases, and a gluten-free diet (GFD) might improve fertility outcomes. However, the general prevalence of infertility in CeD patients does not appear to exceed that of the general population. This review includes evidence on both male and female infertility and examines possible pathophysiological mechanisms, including nutritional deficiencies, immune-mediated effects, and sexual dysfunction. Further high-quality prospective studies are needed to determine the true impact of CeD on reproductive health and to inform screening guidelines.

Keywords: celiac disease; gluten; gluten-free diet; infertility

1. Introduction

Celiac disease (CeD), also known as gluten-sensitive enteropathy, is a chronic immune-mediated enteropathy that occurs in genetically predisposed individuals upon ingestion of gluten, which is found in wheat, rye, barley, and oat products [1]. Pathologically, CeD is characterized by damage to the small-intestinal mucosa, including villous atrophy, crypt hyperplasia, and increased lymphocyte infiltration. The global prevalence of diagnosed CeD is approximately 1%; however, many cases remain undiagnosed, which increases the risk of long-term complications. CeD can affect individuals of any age, both children and adults, with women being at least twice as likely to be affected as men.

Diagnosing CeD is challenging and involves a multi-step process that includes symptom evaluation, serological testing, duodenal biopsy, response to a gluten-free diet (GFD), and, optionally, genetic testing. Due to this complexity, delays in diagnosis, which can sometimes exceed ten years, are common. The only effective treatment currently available is a strict, lifelong GFD, which typically leads to relief of clinical symptoms and healing of small-intestinal damage.

The clinical presentation of CeD is highly variable, ranging from asymptomatic cases to severe symptoms that can be categorized into gastrointestinal and extra-gastrointestinal manifestations. Common gastrointestinal symptoms include chronic diarrhea, abdominal pain, bloating, flatulence, and vomiting [2], which often prompt physicians to initiate diagnostic procedures for CeD. In contrast, extra-gastrointestinal manifestations—such as nutritional deficiencies, bone-related disorders, dental abnormalities, skin conditions, and neurological or psychiatric disorders [3]—are more difficult to detect. Many of these cases remain undiagnosed, particularly in the absence of gastrointestinal symptoms.

Among the extra-intestinal manifestations of CeD, various adverse reproductive outcomes have been reported, including infertility, spontaneous abortion, stillbirth, preterm delivery, and low birth weight [4–8]. Even endocrine conditions like hypogonadotropic hypogonadism, which can lead to infertility, are linked to celiac disease [9–12].

According to the World Health Organization (WHO), overall infertility is defined as the "failure to achieve a clinical pregnancy after 12 months or more of regular unprotected sexual intercourse". Primary infertility refers to the inability to conceive in couples who have never achieved pregnancy, while secondary infertility refers to difficulties in conceiving after previously achieving pregnancy. Unexplained infertility is diagnosed when no apparent cause of infertility can be identified, in both partners, after comprehensive evaluation, but there is no single universally accepted definition of this condition. Unexplained infertility is a diagnosis of exclusion for couples who do not fit the criteria for diagnosis of male factor infertility, oligo/anovulatory infertility or anatomical concerns such as blocked fallopian tubes, endometriosis, uterine cavity defects, or cervical/vaginal obstruction. Primary research studies that recruit couples with unexplained infertility use widely varying inclusion criteria and often do not define their criteria at all [13].

Infertility can stem from female factors, including ovarian, tubal, or endometrial dysfunction, or male factors, such as erectile dysfunction, hypogonadism, or reduced sperm motility. Known causes of infertility include anatomical abnormalities, endocrine disorders, endometriosis, and infections such as Chlamydia trachomatis and tuberculosis. When no identifiable cause is found, an underlying condition such as CeD may be responsible [14,15].

Since the 1970s, numerous studies have explored the association between CeD and infertility. Wang et al. [16] described at least one autoimmune disease in 25% of women with primary ovarian insufficiency with an increased relative risk for CeD of 7.58 [3.47, 14.39]; $p = 4.47 \times 10^{-6}$). However, the findings remain inconsistent, leaving this issue open to debate.

The aim of this review is to summarize recent studies on the relationship between CeD and infertility to raise awareness among physicians about the potential presence of CeD in patients experiencing reproductive difficulties. Numerous studies have explored the association between CeD and infertility; however, the findings remain inconsistent. Previous reviews have focused predominantly on female infertility or have presented limited updates on newer evidence [17]. This review differs by including studies up to July 2024 and analyzing findings across genders and couples, thereby providing a broader perspective. It also aims to highlight inconsistencies and identify knowledge gaps, offering a critical narrative rather than a meta-analytic synthesis.

2. Materials and Methods

PubMed Search Strategy and Selection Criteria

This is a narrative review. A search of the PubMed database was conducted for articles published in English between 2011 and March 2025. The keywords used were "c(o)eliac disease" combined with "infertility" and "fertility". Articles without abstracts, such as case reports, commentaries, conference papers, and letters, were excluded. The initial search identified 84 articles, of which 29 were selected for this review. Additionally, 13 papers were identified through cross-referencing the retrieved articles. We conducted a similar search on Scopus, initially identifying 73 articles in English on fertility and celiac disease; among them, we selected 36 publications: a total of 23 were already included in the PubMed search, while 13 were not. Therefore, we added data from these 13 studies to our review (Figure 1).

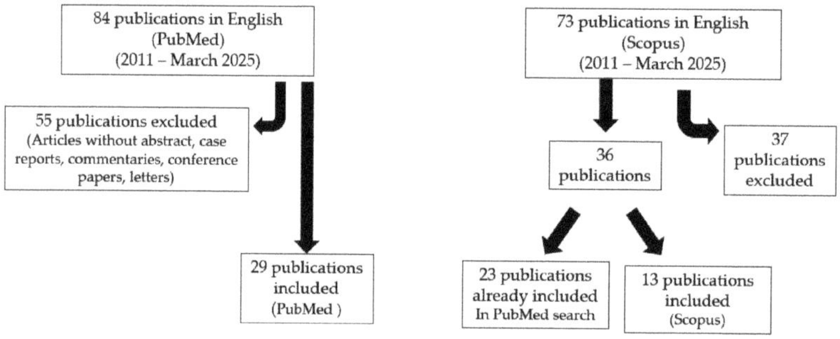

Figure 1. PRISMA flow diagram of search procedure.

3. Results

In 1970, Morris and colleagues were the first to describe the relationship between untreated CeD and female infertility, as well as the impact of a GFD. They reported three cases of infertile women with untreated CeD who successfully conceived after adopting a GFD [18]. Since then, numerous clinical studies have explored the association between CeD and infertility, but their findings have been inconsistent [4,6–8,19].

Several factors may explain the variability in study results, including differences in how CeD (seropositive vs. biopsy-confirmed) and infertility (WHO definition vs. referral to infertility clinics) were defined, as well as variations in the sample sizes and demographic compositions of study populations and control groups. The limited number of participants in most studies (typically fewer than 200) reduces the statistical power of the findings. Additionally, inconsistent data interpretation and a lack of differentiation between overall infertility and unexplained infertility have contributed to the conflicting results. In cases of explained infertility, the underlying causes were rarely detailed.

Screening for undiagnosed CeD among infertile individuals was primarily conducted using serological tests for antibodies against transglutaminase 2 (TGA), endomysium (EMA), and/or gliadin (AGA). However, confirmation of CeD through duodenal biopsy was infrequent.

An overview of relevant clinical studies, published from 2011 to March 2025, is presented in the following subsections. They include the association between CeD and infertility of women, men, and couples and discuss possible pathophysiological mechanisms and the role of a GFD. TGA measurement as a screening method for CeD was the only suitable basis for the comparison of results.

3.1. *Infertility in Women*

To date, the precise risk estimate of infertility in women with CeD remains unclear due to methodological variations and heterogeneity across studies. Furthermore, the impact of a GFD on infertility has not been fully clarified. Findings published before 2011 were reviewed by Lasa et al. [20] and Tersigni et al. [21]. These reviews indicated that undiagnosed CeD appears to be a significant risk factor for infertility in women, and screening for CeD should be considered in cases of unexplained infertility.

Subsequent investigations into the association between CeD and infertility in women have also produced contradictory results.

Table 1 summarizes the prevalence of TGA-positivity among women with overall infertility and unexplained infertility compared to fertile control women.

3.1.1. Positive Associations

Several studies investigating the prevalence of undiagnosed CeD in women with fertility problems have identified a clear association.

A prospective cohort study conducted at an academic infertility clinic in the United States [22] included 188 infertile women, 51 of whom had unexplained infertility (27%). All participants underwent serological screening. Among the 188 women with overall infertility, 3 (1.6%) tested positive for TGA. The expected prevalence of CeD in a similarly aged female population from the same geographical region was 1.3%. However, in a subgroup analysis of women with unexplained infertility, the prevalence rose to 3.9% (2 out of 51 patients).

In a cross-sectional study conducted in India, 230 women with unexplained infertility diagnosed according to WHO criteria 1993, considering normal semen analysis from the partner, and 305 control women were tested for seropositivity [23]. Elevated TGA levels were found in 13 women with unexplained infertility (5.7%) and 4 controls (1.3%), a statistically significant difference ($p = 0.004$). This indicated a 4.5-fold higher prevalence of CeD in infertile women compared to controls. Interestingly, none of the TGA-positive women exhibited classic gastrointestinal symptoms of CeD. The authors concluded that women with unexplained infertility might have subclinical CeD detectable through serological screening.

A Brazilian cross-sectional study of 170 infertile women, including 29 with unexplained infertility, reported a seropositive CeD prevalence of 2.9% (5 out of 170) in the overall cohort and 10.3% (3 out of 29) in the unexplained infertility group [24]. The authors suggested that these findings support the implementation of serological screening for CeD in women with unexplained infertility.

Similarly, a case-control study in Mexico evaluated 171 women with fertility disorders and 171 fertile control women matched by age for CeD-specific antibodies [25]. The results showed that seven infertile patients (4.1%) and only one control woman (0.6%) tested positive for elevated TGA levels.

Two studies from Iran provided additional insights into the prevalence of CeD among infertile women. In one study, serum samples from 100 couples with unexplained infertility and 200 fertile control couples were tested for TGA antibodies [19]. Positive TGA was detected in seven infertile women (7%) and seven control women (3.5%). Another prospective study involving 100 couples with unexplained infertility found that eight women (8%) tested positive for TGA, a prevalence higher than that observed in the general population [26]. Based on these findings, the authors recommended screening all women with unexplained infertility for CeD.

In summary, the results on the prevalence of CeD in women with overall or unexplained infertility revealed that 43 out of 959 (4.5%) had a positive TGA serology (six studies) in comparison to 676 control cases with 12 seropositive women (1.8%) (three studies). In case of unexplained infertility, 30 out of 481 subjects (6.2%) had a positive TGA serology. These findings indicated a significantly increased risk of seropositive CeD in women with infertility and advised that patients with unexplained infertility, particularly, should be screened for CeD.

Another Iranian study, where 8/100 females with infertility tested positive for CeD serology, showed a significant association between high levels of Anti-TTG Ab and infertility (odds ratio = 17.30, 95% CI: 2.13–140.39) [27].

A cross-sectional study conducted in China [28], which collected clinical and biochemical data from a total of 67 females with CeD and 67 healthy patients, showed significantly lower levels of anti-Müllerian hormone and higher Prolactin levels in the CeD group (all $p < 0.05$).

A nationwide Danish matched cohort study [29] involving 6319 women diagnosed with CeD and 63166 controls showed that prior to being diagnosed, CeD women had an excess risk of spontaneous abortion and extra stillbirths per 1000 pregnancies compared with the non-CeD women, indicating that that undiagnosed CeD can affect female reproduction.

The meta-analysis conducted by Singh et al. [30], which included nine studies published up to 2014, found that the prevalence of CeD in women with overall infertility (n = 884) was 2.3%, while the prevalence in women with unexplained infertility (n = 623) was 3.2%. Women with overall infertility were 3.5 times more likely, and those with unexplained infertility were 6 times more likely, to have CeD compared to fertile controls.

Another meta-analysis by Castano et al. [6] reviewed data from 23 scientific articles published up to 2019. The analysis reported similar prevalence rates of CeD-specific serology in women with overall infertility (n = 5935) and those with unexplained infertility (n = 1982), with pooled proportions ranging from approximately 1.3% to 1.6%. This represented a 3-fold increase in the odds of CeD in infertile women compared to the control population (n = 7202). Collectively, the findings of both meta-analyses confirm a higher risk of CeD in infertile women, particularly in those with unexplained infertility.

Conversely, two studies have demonstrated a higher prevalence of infertility in women with untreated CeD. Fortunato et al. [31] evaluated the fertility risk in 4070 women with CeD living in two regions of Southern Italy using ad hoc data and statistics that were routinely collected. They compared the frequency of hospital admissions for fertility issues in these women with 19,765 matched controls without CeD residing in the same region. The proportion of women hospitalized for fertility-related problems was significantly higher among those with CeD compared to age-matched controls (1.2% vs. 0.2%; $p < 0.01$).

In a more recent case-control study conducted in India between 2020 and 2021, Prasad et al. [32] used a detailed questionnaire to evaluate reproductive functions in 288 female patients with biopsy-confirmed CeD. They also included 586 age-matched healthy female controls. The study revealed that women with CeD had a significantly higher rate of current infertility compared to controls (10.5% vs. 5.2%; $p = 0.028$).

Lastly, a retrospective cohort study based on an online survey found higher rates of spontaneous abortion (50.6% vs. 40.6%; $p = 0.01$) and premature delivery (23.6% vs. 15.9%; $p = 0.02$) in women with celiac disease compared to controls [33].

3.1.2. Negative Associations

The following six studies did not find a greater likelihood of CeD in women with infertility compared to controls or the general population.

In a large prospective cohort study conducted in the United States, 995 women undergoing in vitro fertilization were screened for CeD using a specific questionnaire and serological testing [34]. Among the participants, 24 patients (2.4%) tested positive for TGA. This prevalence was not significantly different from that observed in the general population (2.8%).

Another study enrolled 685 women at a Canadian fertility clinic to investigate the prevalence of CeD in women with unexplained infertility versus those with an identifiable cause of infertility [35]. Women on a GFD or with a previous CeD diagnosis were excluded. Eight of the 685 infertile women (1.2%) were identified as seropositive for CeD, including 4 out of 326 women with unexplained infertility (1.2%) and 4 out of 359 women with a known cause of infertility (1.1%). The study concluded that CeD was no more common in women with unexplained infertility than in those with a known infertility cause.

A study conducted in Iran examined 150 women with unexplained infertility and 150 control women for TGA serum levels [36]. Seropositive CeD was identified in three infertile patients (2.0%) and none of the controls, but the difference was not statistically significant ($p = 0.49$).

Three additional studies of infertile couples visiting fertility clinics provided further insight into the frequency of CeD in women. Hogen Esch et al. [37] screened 1038 subfertile male–female couples in the Netherlands for IgA TGA and IgA EMA. The prevalence of seropositive CeD among the women was 0.6% (6 out of 1038), which was not significantly higher than in the general Dutch population.

In a prospective pilot study, 65 Turkish couples with unexplained infertility were examined for CeD-specific antibodies, including TGA [38]. None of the women tested positive for any of the CeD-specific antibodies.

Finally, a cross-sectional study in Denmark estimated the prevalence of unrecognized CeD among infertile couples using TGA testing [39]. Among the 455 participating women, 4 (0.9%) were antibody-positive, comparable to the Danish general population.

In summary, these six studies revealed that among 3388 women with overall or unexplained infertility, 44 subjects (1.3%) had a positive TGA serology, which appears to be not higher than that of the general population. This finding did not support the routine screening of women with infertility for CeD. Only one of these studies included a control group, and none of the participating 150 subjects was seropositive [36].

A recent systematic review with meta-analysis of the prevalence of CeD in women with infertility also demonstrated that the prevalence of CeD in infertile women was not increased compared with controls [40]. Overall, 20 studies, published until February 2020, were included in the analysis. Based on 11 studies (1617 women), the pooled prevalence of biopsy-confirmed CeD was 0.7% in women with overall infertility. Restricting the study population to women with unexplained infertility, the pooled prevalence of biopsy-confirmed CeD was 0.6%. Regarding studies where CeD had been defined per serology (20 studies; 5158 women), the pooled prevalence of CeD was 1.1% in women with any infertility. In conclusion, results indicated that the prevalence of CeD was not higher in infertile women compared with the general population.

Vice versa, two investigations examined the prevalence of infertility in women with CeD. A large population-based study from the United Kingdom included 2,426,225 women of child-bearing age; 6506 women (0.3%) had a diagnosis of CeD [41]. The results revealed that the rate of infertility among women with CeD (4.4%) was similar to that of women without CeD (4.1%). As an exception, the rate was significantly higher among women diagnosed with CeD when they were 25–29 years old compared with women in the same age group without CeD. A Slovenian retrospective case-control study, including 205 women with biopsy-confirmed CeD and 103 healthy women, demonstrated that 23 subjects with CeD (11.2%) reported being treated for infertility, which was not statistically significant ($p = 0.425$) when compared with 8 control subjects (7.8%) [42].

A recent Italian survey of 493 celiac women revealed links between untreated celiac disease and miscarriages, anemia, low birth weight, and infertility; 73% felt poorly informed by healthcare professionals about reproductive risks [43].

Nahan et al. [44] identified >25,000,000 outpatient women without CeD, and 9368 with CeD from the database of 80 healthcare organisations. They reported that women with CeD had higher odds of later women's health conditions including absent/rare menstruation (4.6% vs. 2.0%; OR 2.34), infertility (1.4% vs. 0.9%; OR 1.69), polycystic ovarian syndrome

(3.3% vs. 1.0%; OR 3.2), menopausal disorders (4.3% vs. 1.56%; OR 285), and primary ovarian failure (0.96% vs. 0.16%; OR 6.25).

Mendelian randomization analysis, including data from 12,041 CD cases and 12,228 controls, from 14,759 infertile women, and from 111,583 controls, obtained from FinnGen and UK Biobank databases, revealed that there was no discernible link between genetic susceptibility to CD and female infertility [45]. The authors concluded that this finding implied a restrained basis for advocating CeD screening among women facing infertility issues.

Several studies and meta-analyses demonstrated a trend towards an increased prevalence of CeD in women with infertility and, vice versa, of infertility in women with active CeD, particularly in cases of unexplained infertility. Other investigations indicated that CeD is not more common in infertile women than in the general population. Figure 2 summarizes the results of a selection of studies about female infertility. All the papers published have some strengths and limitations. Screening for CeD in infertile women has been judged in a variety of different ways, and a widespread consensus is lacking. Further targeted prospective studies are needed to investigate the association between CeD and infertility in women.

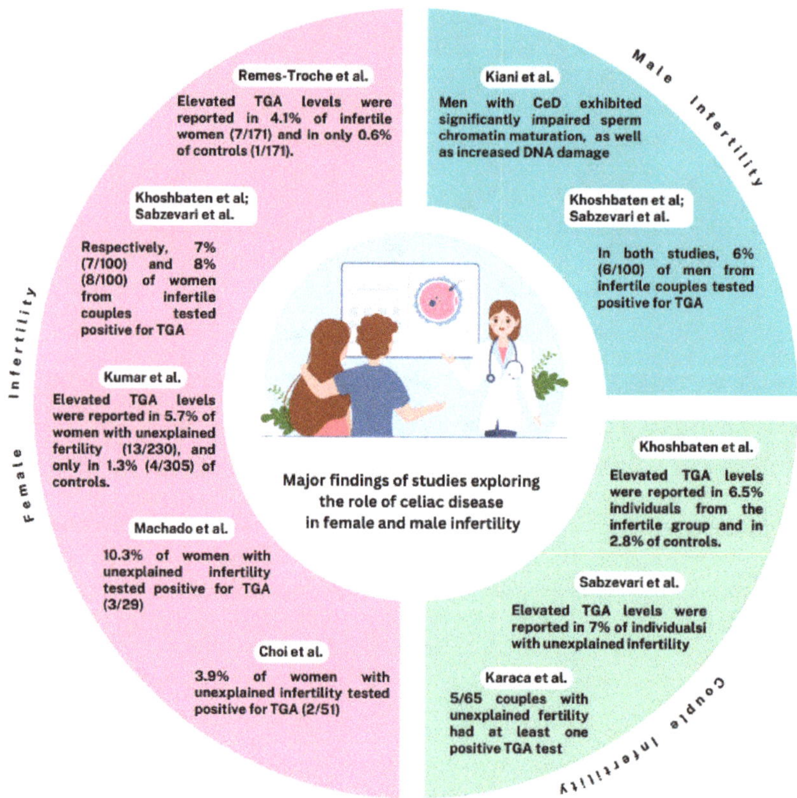

Figure 2. A selection of studies about CeD and female, male, and couple infertility.

Table 1. Frequency of TGA-positive women with overall and unexplained infertility compared with fertile controls.

Author (Year) [Ref.]	Country [a]	Overall Infertility		Unexplained Infertility		Controls	
		n [b]	TGA (%)	n [b]	TGA (%)	n [b]	TGA (%)
Choi (2011) [22]	US	188	3 (1.6)	51	2 (3.9)	-	-
Hogen Esch (2011) [37]	NL	1038	6 (0.6)	-	-	-	-
Khoshbaten (2011) [19]	IR	-	-	100	7 (7.0)	200	7 (3.5)
Kumar (2011) [23]	IN	-	-	230	13 (5.7)	305	4 (1.3)
Machado (2013) [24]	BR	170	5 (2.9)	29	3 (10.3)	-	-
Karaca (2015) [38]	TR	-	-	65	0 (0.0)	-	-
Sabzevari (2017) [26]	IR	-	-	100	8 (8.0)	-	-
Grode (2018) [29]	DN	455	4 (0.9)	-	-	-	-
Gunn (2018) [35]	CA	685	8 (1.2)	326	4 (1.2)	-	-
Juneau (2018) [34]	US	995	24 (2.4)	-	-	-	-
Farzaneh (2019) [36]	IR	-	-	150	3 (2.0)	150	0 (0.0)
Remes-Troche (2023) [25]	MX	171	7 (4.1)	-	-	171	1 (0.6)

[a] Country code ISO 3166-1. [b] Number of subjects. Legend: TGA: tissue transglutaminase antibodies; US: United States; NL: Netherlands, IR: Iran, IN: India, BR: Brazil, TR: Turkey, DN: Denmark, CA: Canada, MX: Mexico.

3.2. *Infertility in Men*

The underlying causes of infertility in men with CeD remain unclear and may involve multiple factors. A significant aspect of this increased infertility is represented by abnormalities in sperm parameters, including concentration, motility, and morphology. Beyond the general malabsorption observed in patients with active CeD, deficiencies in essential elements such as selenium and zinc are potential contributors to male infertility. Zinc, for instance, plays a critical role in various stages of sperm development, from germ cell maturation to the spermiation process [46]. Therefore, evaluating selenium and zinc levels in male patients with CeD who are experiencing infertility could be a valuable component of preconception counseling. Oxidative stress has been identified as another key factor in male infertility, contributing to lower sperm functionality. Figure 1 summarizes the results of a selection of studies about male infertility. A case-control study conducted in Iran investigated this phenomenon by comparing semen samples collected from 11 fertile men without CeD and 10 men affected by CeD [47]. The findings indicated that men with CeD exhibited significantly impaired sperm chromatin maturation, characterized by persistent histones and protamine deficiency, as well as increased DNA damage, compared to fertile controls ($p < 0.05$). Furthermore, the sperm viability percentage was significantly lower in men with CeD than in fertile controls ($p < 0.05$).

Studies regarding the fertility of men with CeD are relatively scarce. In 2011, Zugna et al. [48] assessed the fertility in a Swedish cohort of 7121 men with biopsy-confirmed CeD (Marsh type 3). The study group was compared with 31,677 men without CeD matched for age. The number of their children was the main outcome measure of the study. Results showed that men with CeD had a total of 9935 children, averaging 1.40 children per man, compared to 42,245 children, or 1.33 per man, in the control group. Furthermore, approximately 38% of men with CeD had no offspring, a proportion comparable to the reference population (39%). The study concluded that men with diagnosed CeD exhibit normal fertility rates.

Five studies that investigated the prevalence of CeD in couples with reproductive complications (see Section 3.3) provided information about infertility of male participants with CeD. In one of these studies, serum samples were analyzed from 100 Iranian couples with unexplained infertility [19]. As a comparison, 200 couples with no reported reproductive issues and at least one uncomplicated birth served as the control group. TGA were detected in six men (6%) from the study group and four men (4%) from the control group.

In another Iranian study, also including 100 couples with unexplained infertility, participants were tested for TGA serum levels [26]. In patients with positive serologic tests, a duodenal biopsy was performed to confirm the diagnosis. Overall, six men (6%) had positive TGA, and CeD was verified by duodenal biopsy in four subjects.

While both studies revealed a higher prevalence of CeD compared to the general population, neither was statistically significant.

In contrast, the other three studies did not find an association between infertility and CeD. Hogen Esch et al. [37] determined the prevalence of unrecognized CeD in 1038 subfertile male–female couples by testing IgA TGA and IgA EMA levels. Four men (0.4%) tested positive, a rate which was not higher than that of the adult population of the Netherlands. A total of 65 Turkish couples with unexplained infertility were tested for TGA and other CeD-specific antibodies [38]. Only one male partner (1.5%) was seropositive, and histological findings were compatible with Marsh type 3a. Screening for CeD in Danish couples with fertility problems, using TGA testing, revealed that 4 out of 438 men (0.9%) were antibody-positive [39]. CeD was confirmed by biopsy in three men. The prevalence of unrecognized CeD was equivalent to that of the Danish adult population. Altogether, further comprehensive studies should clarify the association between male infertility and CeD.

3.3. *Infertility in Couples*

A large cohort study conducted in the Netherlands investigated the prevalence of undiagnosed CeD in 1038 subfertile male–female couples attending a fertility clinic. Screening was performed using IgA TGA and IgA EMA [37]. The overall prevalence of CeD in this cohort was 0.48% (six females and four males), which was not significantly higher than the general adult population prevalence in the Netherlands (0.35%). Additionally, no significant association was found between CeD and subfertility between genders.

Another study, conducted in Iran, assessed serum samples from 100 couples with unexplained infertility to evaluate the prevalence of CeD [19]. The control group consisted of 200 couples without reproductive complications who had delivered at least one uncomplicated birth. Positive results of TGA were detected in 13 individuals from the infertile group (6.5%) and in 11 controls (2.8%), with a statistically significant difference ($p = 0.027$). The odds ratio (OR) for CeD in couples with unexplained infertility was 2.39, indicating a significantly higher seroprevalence of CeD in the infertile group compared to the fertile controls.

In a study involving 65 Turkish couples with unexplained infertility who were admitted to a fertility clinic, participants were tested for TGA and other CeD-specific antibodies [38]. Endoscopy was performed in patients with positive serology. Five couples had at least one positive antibody test; however, no couple showed antibody positivity in both partners simultaneously. Among the male participants, only one tested positive for all the antibodies. Histopathological examination of the antibody-positive patients revealed that only this male participant showed findings consistent with Marsh type 3a. Ultimately, a diagnosis of CeD was confirmed in only one couple (1.5%), with no female patients being diagnosed with CeD.

A prospective cross-sectional study from Iran included 100 couples with unexplained infertility who were tested for TGA levels [26]. In patients with positive serologic tests, a duodenal biopsy was performed to confirm the diagnosis. Overall, 14 patients (7%) with unexplained infertility had positive TGA (8 women and 6 men). In 11 out of 200 patients (5.5%), endoscopic finding was compatible with biopsy-verified CeD (7 women, 4 men).

A cross-sectional study was conducted to estimate the prevalence of unrecognized CeD among Danish couples referred for fertility treatment. Screening involved TGA testing, followed by small-bowel biopsies to confirm the diagnosis [39]. Out of 893 participants (51% women), 4 men and 4 women (0.90%) tested positive for TGA. Small-bowel biopsies were performed on seven seropositive individuals, corresponding to an overall prevalence of 0.45%. The prevalence of unrecognized CeD was equivalent to that of the Danish general population (0.48%).

Overall, two studies showed a positive association between infertility of couples and CeD: Around 7% of 200 couples reported problems with infertility [19,26]. In contrast, three studies did not find any significant relation. Only 0.5–1.5% of couples with reproductive problems were identified to have CeD, which corresponded to the general population [37–39]. Figure 2 summarizes the results of a selection of studies about couple infertility. Further investigations to address this issue are required.

4. Pathophysiological Mechanism

The etiology of infertility in CeD is multifactorial and remains only partially understood. Two main mechanisms have been proposed: micronutrient deficiencies and immune–endocrine dysregulation.

Micronutrient malabsorption is common in untreated CeD and includes iron, folate, selenium, zinc, and fat-soluble vitamins. These elements are crucial for gametogenesis, ovulation, implantation, and fetal development [49]. Zinc and selenium, in particular, influence sperm maturation and endometrial receptivity.

Immune-mediated and endocrine factors may further compromise reproductive health. Autoantibodies such as TGAs and anti-thyroid antibodies, as well as increased pro-inflammatory cytokines (e.g., IL-6, TNF-α), can impair endometrial angiogenesis and placentation. Hormonal disturbances, including altered prolactin, FSH, and LH levels, have also been observed [50,51].

Moreover, CeD is associated with menstrual irregularities, delayed menarche, and early menopause, possibly narrowing the reproductive window [52]. In men, oxidative stress and sexual dysfunction—including erectile and ejaculation disorders—may also contribute to reduced fertility.

Sexual dysfunction in women, including decreased sexual desire, dyspareunia (pain during intercourse), and anorgasmia (absence of orgasm), may contribute to infertility in patients with CeD [53]. Additionally, untreated CeD has been associated with delayed menarche and premature menopause, leading to a shorter fertile window compared to women without CeD [54]. In men, increased oxidative stress—a recurring finding in infertile males—has been linked to reduced sperm quality and function. Male infertility factors in CeD may also include erectile dysfunction and impaired sperm parameters, such as reduced quality and motility. Despite these observations, understanding the pathophysiological mechanisms underlying infertility in CeD remains limited, highlighting the need for further research.

5. Effect of a GFD

Morris et al. [18] were the first to report a link between untreated CeD and female infertility, as well as the positive impact of a GFD. They described three cases of infertile women with untreated CeD who conceived after adopting a GFD. Subsequent studies have demonstrated the beneficial effects of a GFD in improving fertility in women with CeD [7]. For instance, Nenna et al. reported four women (aged 28–39 years) in Italy who sought infertility treatment for periods ranging from 2 to 12 years and were subsequently diagnosed with CeD [55]. Remarkably, all four women conceived after adhering to a GFD for 2–9 months. One notable case involved a 39-year-old woman who had unsuccessfully tried to conceive for 11 years, including 4 years undergoing in vitro fertilization who, after following a GFD for 2 years, successfully delivered a baby.

A prospective cohort study conducted at an academic infertility clinic in the USA included 188 infertile women who underwent serologic screening for CeD [20]. Patients with positive serologic tests were advised to confirm the diagnosis with small-intestinal biopsies. Four women were diagnosed with CeD, confirmed by biopsy, and received nutritional counseling to adopt a GFD. Remarkably, all four women conceived within a year following their diagnosis and dietary changes.

In a retrospective study from a Spanish infertility clinic, the impact of a GFD was assessed in women with CeD who had experienced recurrent implantation failure [56]. Data from women following a gluten-containing diet (GCD) were compared with those adhering to a GFD. Significant differences were observed: the live birth rate was 0% (0/19) for women on a GCD versus 60% (6/10) for those on a GFD ($p = 0.004$), and the miscarriage rate was 100% (3/3) for the GCD group compared to 14% (1/7) in the GFD group ($p = 0.033$).

A retrospective study from Morocco demonstrated that reproductive disorders in patients with celiac disease are frequent (58/173 patients) but largely reversible, with 90% of cases (26 patients out of 29) showing improvement following the initiation of a gluten-free diet [57].

However, contrasting results emerged from a USA study of 28 women with seropositive CeD undergoing in vitro fertilization [34]. Outcomes in women adhering to a GFD (n = 3) were comparable to those on a GCD. Parameters such as mature oocytes retrieved (10.2 vs. 10.8), fertilization rates (82.4% vs. 83.6%), and blastulation rates (54.8% vs. 48.6%) showed no significant differences ($p = 0.37$–0.58). A notable limitation of this study, and others, was the lack of rigorous testing for strict GFD adherence.

In conclusion, further investigations involving larger cohorts of CeD patients, including those strictly adherent and non-adherent to a GFD, are required to clarify the role of a GFD in addressing fertility issues in women with CeD.

6. Discussion

Despite decades of research, the association between CeD and infertility remains controversial. Some studies show increased prevalence of CeD among women with unexplained infertility, while others report no difference from the general population. These discrepancies may stem from variability in diagnostic criteria, population characteristics, and methodology.

A limitation of our review is the use only of PubMed and Scopus as a source database, which may have limited the comprehensiveness of the literature search. Furthermore, as a narrative review, study selection and data interpretation are inherently subjective, introducing potential bias. Other limitations in the research include small sample sizes and the absence of control groups.

The prevalence of CeD varies geographically and ethnically, ranging from under 0.1% in East Asia to over 1% in Europe and the Middle East. The low prevalence of CeD in non-Caucasian women may reflect a combination of genetic, diagnostic, and healthcare disparities rather than biological differences. While CeD is more common in white populations due to genetic predisposition [58], underdiagnosis due to limited access to testing in non-Caucasian populations may be exaggerating the disparity. Non-Caucasian women with CeD often depend on community health centers rather than primary care settings, where access to diagnostic tools may be limited. As a result, being female, non-

Caucasian, and having undiagnosed celiac disease likely creates a triple burden, increasing the risk of delayed diagnosis and inadequate care [59].

These disparities must be taken into account when evaluating the clinical utility of screening for CeD in infertile populations. A "one-size-fits-all" approach is not appropriate, and pretest probability should guide testing. Moreover, many studies rely primarily on serological testing without confirming diagnoses through duodenal biopsy. The standard laboratory tests for CeD screening have commonly included IgA TGA, IgA EMA, and total IgA antibodies. In recent years, rapid point-of-care (POC) tests have been proposed as alternatives to standard testing. However, Grode et al. evaluated the diagnostic accuracy of the POC test (Simtomax®) and found it unsuitable due to a high rate of false-positive results (sensitivity = 42.9%) [60].

Another confounding factor is that some studies failed to clearly distinguish between infertility and sexual dysfunction. CeD may not inherently reduce reproductive capacity but associated depression, fatigue, or dyspareunia could affect sexual activity, thereby reducing conception rates.

While routine screening for CeD in infertile patients remains controversial, several studies have demonstrated the positive impact of a GFD on fertility in women with CeD. Adhering to a strict GFD has been shown to improve the chances of conception and the birth of a healthy child. Patients must also be informed of the importance of dietary compliance, as any lapses in following a GFD can significantly reduce their likelihood of achieving a successful outcome [61].

In summary, further studies are required to evaluate the risk of unrecognized CeD in infertile patients to define the role of routine serological screening for CeD in infertile patients and to elucidate the underlying mechanism for infertility in active CeD. Future research should employ standardized infertility definitions; include control groups matched for age, region, and socio-economic status; and use structured protocols (e.g., PRISMA-ScR) with validated tools for bias assessment. Prospective studies that stratify patients by their adherence to a gluten-free diet and by reproductive outcomes are also warranted. Future research should consider the following points: the diagnosis of CeD should include serological standardized testing of TGA, EMA, and total IgA antibodies followed by confirmatory duodenal biopsy (Marsh criteria) in all seropositive patients. The definition of infertility should be based on the WHO definition or a close version. The sample size of participants should be more than 200 infertile patients and 200 controls with proven fertility, the latter being matched for age, socio-economic status, and regional origin.

Author Contributions: Conceptualization, H.W., C.C. and A.S.; methodology, H.W., C.C.; software, C.S.; resources, C.G., L.P.; data curation, C.C., A.S.; writing—original draft preparation, H.W.; writing—review and editing, C.C., A.S.; visualization, C.S., C.G., L.P.; supervision, C.C., A.S. All authors have read and agreed to the published version of the manuscript.

Funding: This research received no external funding.

Data Availability Statement: The original contributions presented in the study are included in the article; further inquiries can be directed to the corresponding author.

Conflicts of Interest: The authors declare no conflicts of interest.

References

1. Catassi, C.; Verdu, E.F.; Bai, J.C.; Lionetti, E. Coeliac disease. *Lancet* **2022**, *399*, 2413–2426. [CrossRef]
2. Wieser, H.; Ciacci, C.; Soldaini, C.; Gizzi, C.; Santonicola, A. Gastrointestinal and Hepatobiliary Manifestations Associated with Untreated Celiac Disease in Adults and Children: A Narrative Overview. *J. Clin. Med.* **2024**, *13*, 4579. [CrossRef] [PubMed]
3. Santonicola, A.; Wieser, H.; Gizzi, C.; Soldaini, C.; Ciacci, C. Associations between Celiac Disease, Extra-Gastrointestinal Manifestations, and Gluten-Free Diet: A Narrative Overview. *Nutrients* **2024**, *16*, 1814. [CrossRef] [PubMed]

4. Casella, G.; Orfanotti, G.; Giacomantonio, L.; Di Bella, C.; Crisafulli, V.; Villanacci, V.; Baldini, V.; Bassotti, G. Celiac disease and obstetrical-gynecological contribution. *Gastroenterol. Hepatol. Bed Bench* **2016**, *9*, 241–249. [PubMed]
5. Saccone, G.; Berghella, V.; Sarno, L.; Maruotti, G.M.; Cetin, I.; Greco, L.; Khashan, A.S.; McCarthy, F.; Martinelli, D.; Fortunato, F.; et al. Celiac disease and obstetric complications: A systematic review and metaanalysis. *Am. J. Obstet. Gynecol.* **2016**, *214*, 225–234. [CrossRef]
6. Castaño, M.; Gómez-Gordo, R.; Cuevas, D.; Núñez, C. Systematic Review and Meta-Analysis of Prevalence of Coeliac Disease in Women with Infertility. *Nutrients* **2019**, *11*, 1950. [CrossRef]
7. Schiepatti, A.; Sprio, E.; Sanders, D.S.; Lovati, E.; Biagi, F. Coeliac disease and obstetric and gynaecological disorders: Where are we now? *Eur. J. Gastroenterol. Hepatol.* **2019**, *31*, 425–433. [CrossRef]
8. Arvanitakis, K.; Siargkas, A.; Germanidis, G.; Dagklis, T.; Tsakiridis, I. Adverse pregnancy outcomes in women with celiac disease: A systematic review and meta-analysis. *Ann. Gastroenterol.* **2023**, *36*, 12–24. [CrossRef]
9. Tønnes Pedersen, A.; Cleemann, L.; Main, K.M.; Juul, A. Transition in Pediatric and Adolescent Hypogonadal Girls: Gynecological Aspects, Estrogen Replacement Therapy, and Contraception. *Endocr. Dev.* **2018**, *33*, 113–127.
10. Galal, M.S.; Musa, S.A.; Babiker, O.O.; Hamdan, H.Z.; Abdullah, M.A. Clinical profile and aetiologies of delayed puberty: A 15 years' experience from a tertiary centre in Sudan. *J. Pediatr. Endocrinol. Metab.* **2022**, *35*, 938–945. [CrossRef]
11. Ergür, A.T.; Öçal, G.; Berberoğlu, M.; Adıyaman, P.; Şıklar, Z.; Aycan, Z.; Evliyaoğlu, O.; Kansu, A.; Girgin, N.; Ensari, A. Celiac disease and autoimmune thyroid disease in children with type 1 diabetes mellitus: Clinical and hla-genotyping results-original article. *J. Clin. Res. Pediatr. Endocrinol.* **2010**, *2*, 151–154. [CrossRef]
12. Walker, M.D.; Zylberberg, H.M.; Green, P.H.R.; Katz, M.S. Endocrine complications of celiac disease: A case report and review of the literature. *Endocr. Res.* **2019**, *44*, 27–45. [CrossRef] [PubMed]
13. Raperport, C.; Desai, J.; Qureshi, D.; Rustin, E.; Balaji, A.; Chronopoulou, E.; Homburg, R.; Khan, K.S.; Bhide, P. The definition of unexplained infertility: A systematic review. *BJOG Int. J. Obstet. Gynaecol.* **2024**, *131*, 880–897. [CrossRef] [PubMed]
14. Hart, R.J. Physiological Aspects of Female Fertility: Role of the Environment, Modern Lifestyle, and Genetics. *Physiol. Rev.* **2016**, *96*, 873–909. [CrossRef] [PubMed]
15. Peterson, M.; Grossman, S. Managing Celiac Disease for Women: Implications for the Primary Care Provider. *Gastroenterol. Nurs. Off. J. Soc. Gastroenterol. Nurses Assoc.* **2016**, *39*, 186–194. [CrossRef] [PubMed]
16. Wang, V.; AWalsh, J.; Zell, J.; EVerrilli, L.; Letourneau, J.M.; Johnstone, E.B.; Allen-Brady, K.; Welt, C.K. Autoimmune Disease is Increased in Women with Primary Ovarian Insufficiency. *J. Clin. Endocrinol. Metab.* **2024**, dgae828. [CrossRef]
17. Olivera, P.; Lasa, J. Celiac Disease and the Risk of Infertility. *Int. J. Celiac Dis.* **2015**, *3*, 84–86. [CrossRef]
18. Morris, J.S.; Adjukiewicz, A.B.; Read, A.E. Coeliac infertility: An indication for dietary gluten restriction? *Lancet* **1970**, *1*, 213–214. [CrossRef]
19. Khoshbaten, M.; Rostami Nejad, M.; Farzady, L.; Sharifi, N.; Hashemi, S.H.; Rostami, K. Fertility disorder associated with celiac disease in males and females: Fact or fiction? *J. Obstet. Gynaecol. Res.* **2011**, *37*, 1308–1312. [CrossRef]
20. Lasa, J.S.; Zubiaurre, I.; Soifer, L.O. Risk of infertility in patients with celiac disease: A meta-analysis of observational studies. *Arq. Gastroenterol.* **2014**, *51*, 144–150. [CrossRef]
21. Tersigni, C.; Castellani, R.; de Waure, C.; Fattorossi, A.; De Spirito, M.; Gasbarrini, A.; Scambia, G.; Di Simone, N. Celiac disease and reproductive disorders: Meta-analysis of epidemiologic associations and potential pathogenic mechanisms. *Hum. Reprod. Updat.* **2014**, *20*, 582–593. [CrossRef] [PubMed]
22. Choi, J.M.; Lebwohl, B.; Wang, J.; Lee, S.K.; AMurray, J.; Sauer, M.V.; Green, P.H.R. Increased prevalence of celiac disease in patients with unexplained infertility in the United States. *J. Reprod. Med.* **2011**, *56*, 199–203. [PubMed]
23. Kumar, A.; Meena, M.; Begum, N.; Kumar, N.; Gupta, R.K.; Aggarwal, S.; Prasad, S.; Batra, S. Latent celiac disease in reproductive performance of women. *Fertil. Steril.* **2011**, *95*, 922–927. [CrossRef]
24. Machado, A.P.D.S.L.; Silva, L.R.; Zausner, B.; Oliveira, J.D.A.; Diniz, D.R.; De Oliveira, J. Undiagnosed celiac disease in women with infertility. *J. Reprod. Med.* **2013**, *58*, 61–66. [PubMed]
25. Remes-Troche, J.M.; Sánchez-Vargas, L.A.; Ríos-Gálvez, S.; Cano-Contreras, A.D.; Amerena-Abreu, J.; Cruz-Patiño, E.; Meixueiro-Daza, A.; Vivanco-Cid, H. Celiac disease seroprevalence in patients with infertility. A case-control study. *Gac. Medica Mexico* **2023**, *159*, 142–146. [CrossRef]
26. Sabzevari, A.; Yazdanbod, A.; Aghdam, F.K.; Maleki, N. Prevalence of celiac disease among iranian couples with unexplained infertility: A prospective study. *J. Reprod. Med.* **2017**, *62*, 659–664.
27. Rahimpour, E.; Shojaei-Zarghani, S.; Amooee, S.; Safarpour, A.; Geramizadeh, B.; Zahmatkeshan, M. The Frequency of Celiac Disease and Its Association with Infertility in Women Attending Infertility Clinics: A Case-Control Study in Southern Iran. *Shiraz E-Med. J.* **2024**, *25*, e145384. [CrossRef]
28. Tuerxuntayi, A.; Shi, T.; Gao, B.; Feng, Y.; Li, T.; Hui, W.; Xue, S.; Gao, F. Serum anti-mullerian hormone, sex hormone, and nutrient levels in reproductive age women with celiac disease. *J. Assist. Reprod. Genet.* **2024**, *41*, 2129–2136. [CrossRef]

29. Grode, L.; Bech, B.H.; Plana-Ripoll, O.; Bliddal, M.; Agerholm, I.E.; Humaidan, P.; Ramlau-Hansen, C.H. Reproductive life in women with celiac disease: A nationwide, population-based matched cohort study. *Hum. Reprod.* **2018**, *33*, 1538–1547. [CrossRef]
30. Singh, P.; Arora, S.; Lal, S.; Strand, T.A.; Makharia, G.K. Celiac Disease in Women with Infertility: A meta-Analysis. *J. Clin. Gastroenterol.* **2016**, *50*, 33–39. [CrossRef]
31. Fortunato, F.; Martinelli, D.; Prato, R.; Pedalino, B. Results from ad hoc and routinely collected data among celiac women with infertility or pregnancy related disorders: Italy, 2001–2011. *Sci. World J.* **2014**, *2014*, 614269. [CrossRef]
32. Prasad, S.; Singh, P.; Singh, A.; Mehtab, W.; Rajput, S.; Dang, S.; Chauhan, A.; Rajput, M.S.; Kachhawa, G.; Jagannath, S.; et al. Reproductive functions and pregnancy outcome in female patients with celiac disease. *J. Gastroenterol. Hepatol.* **2024**, *39*, 1310–1317. [CrossRef] [PubMed]
33. Moleski, S.M.; Lindenmeyer, C.C.; Veloski, J.J.; Miller, R.S.; Miller, C.L.; Kastenberg, D.; DiMarino, A.J. Increased rates of pregnancy complications in women with celiac disease. *Ann. Gastroenterol.* **2015**, *28*, 236–240. [PubMed]
34. Juneau, C.R.; Franasiak, J.M.; Goodman, L.R.; Marin, D.; Scott, K.; Morin, S.J.; Neal, S.A.; Juneau, J.E.; Scott, R.T. Celiac disease is not more prevalent in patients undergoing in vitro fertilization and does not affect reproductive outcomes with or without treatment: A large prospective cohort study. *Fertil. Steril.* **2018**, *110*, 437–442. [CrossRef] [PubMed]
35. Gunn, B.; Murphy, K.E.; Greenblatt, E.M. Unexplained Infertility and Undiagnosed Celiac Disease: Study of a Multiethnic Canadian Population. *J. Obstet. Gynaecol. Can.* **2018**, *40*, 293–298. [CrossRef]
36. Farzaneh, F.; Khalili, M. Prevalence of Celiac in Fertile Women Due to Unexplained Infertility. *La Prensa Medica Argent.* **2019**, *105*, 4. [CrossRef]
37. Esch, C.E.H.; Van Rijssen, M.J.; Roos, A.; Koning, F.; Dekker, F.W.; Mearin, M.L.; Helmerhorst, F.M.; Schweizer, J.J. Screening for unrecognized coeliac disease in subfertile couples. *Scand. J. Gastroenterol.* **2011**, *46*, 1423–1428. [CrossRef]
38. Karaca, N.; Yılmaz, R.; Aktun, L.H.; Batmaz, G.; Karaca, Ç. Is there any relationship between unrecognized Celiac disease and unexplained infertile couples? *Turk. J. Gastroenterol.* **2015**, *26*, 484–486. [CrossRef]
39. Grode, L.B.; EAgerholm, I.; Humaidan, P.; Parkner, T.; Bech, B.H.; Ramlau-Hansen, C.H.; Jensen, T.M. Unrecognised coeliac disease among men and women undergoing fertility treatment: A screening study. *United Eur. Gastroenterol. J.* **2018**, *6*, 1477–1484. [CrossRef]
40. Glimberg, I.; Haggård, L.; Lebwohl, B.; Green, P.H.R.; Ludvigsson, J.F. The prevalence of celiac disease in women with infertility—A systematic review with meta-analysis. *Reprod. Med. Biol.* **2021**, *20*, 224–233. [CrossRef]
41. Dhalwani, N.N.; West, J.; Sultan, A.A.; Ban, L.; Tata, L.J. Women with celiac disease present with fertility problems no more often than women in the general population. *Gastroenterology* **2014**, *147*, 1267–1274.e1. [CrossRef]
42. Pogačar, M.Š.; Vlaisavljević, V.; Turk, E.; Mičetić-Turk, D. Reproductive complications in celiac disease patients in Slovenia. *Eur. J. Obstet. Gynecol. Reprod. Biol.* **2019**, *238*, 90–94. [CrossRef]
43. Arcieri, M.; Abrami, C.; Graziano, A.; Restaino, S.; Barbui, E.; Rizzante, E.; D'ippolito, S.; Vizzielli, G.; Driul, L. The influence of celiac disease on fertility and pregnancy: An Italian survey. *Arch. Gynecol. Obstet.* **2024**, *310*, 2907–2914. [CrossRef]
44. Nanah, R.; Jansson-Knodell, C.; Chatterjee, A.; Nanah, R.; Nanah, M.H.; Almasri, J.; Ford, A.; Hamid, O.; Telbany, A.; Rubio-Tapia, A. Women's Health Disorders in a Coeliac Disease Population After Diagnosis—A Nationwide Cohort Analysis. *Aliment. Pharmacol. Ther.* **2025**, *61*, 1603–1611. [CrossRef] [PubMed]
45. Yuan, S.; Chen, J.; Li, X.; Leffler, D.A.; Larsson, S.C.; Ludvigsson, J.F. No association between celiac disease and female infertility: Evidence from Mendelian randomization analysis. *Fertil. Steril.* **2024**, *122*, 1144–1146. [CrossRef] [PubMed]
46. Foresta, C.; Garolla, A.; Cosci, I.; Menegazzo, M.; Ferigo, M.; Gandin, V.; De Toni, L. Role of zinc trafficking in male fertility: From germ to sperm. *Hum. Reprod.* **2014**, *29*, 1134–1145. [CrossRef] [PubMed]
47. Kiani, S.; Tavalaee, M.; Maghool, F.; Jamali, N.; Emami, M.H.; Nasr-Esfahani, M.H. Sperm Parameters and Chromatin Integrity in Men Suffering from Celiac Disease: Insights into Reproductive Health, Case-Control Study. *Cell J.* **2024**, *26*, 202–209. [CrossRef]
48. Zugna, D.; Richiardi, L.; Akre, O.; Stephansson, O.; Ludvigsson, J.F. Celiac disease is not a risk factor for infertility in men. *Fertil. Steril.* **2011**, *95*, 1709–1713.e3. [CrossRef]
49. Gernand, A.D.; Schulze, K.J.; Stewart, C.P.; West, K.P., Jr.; Christian, P. Micronutrient deficiencies in pregnancy worldwide: Health effects and prevention. *Nat. Rev. Endocrinol.* **2016**, *12*, 274–289. [CrossRef]
50. Sóñora, C.; Calo, G.; Fraccaroli, L.; Pérez-Leirós, C.; Hernández, A.; Ramhorst, R. Tissue transglutaminase on trophoblast cells as a possible target of autoantibodies contributing to pregnancy complications in celiac patients. *Am. J. Reprod. Immunol.* **2014**, *72*, 485–495. [CrossRef]
51. Di Simone, N.; Gratta, M.; Castellani, R.; D'ippolito, S.; Specchia, M.; Scambia, G.; Tersigni, C. Celiac disease and reproductive failures: An update on pathogenic mechanisms. *Am. J. Reprod. Immunol.* **2021**, *85*, e13334. [CrossRef] [PubMed]
52. Freeman, H.J. Reproductive changes associated with celiac disease. *World J. Gastroenterol.* **2010**, *16*, 5810–5814. [CrossRef] [PubMed]

53. Romano, L.; Pellegrino, R.; Sciorio, C.; Barone, B.; Gravina, A.G.; Santonastaso, A.; Mucherino, C.; Astretto, S.; Napolitano, L.; Aveta, A.; et al. Erectile and sexual dysfunction in male and female patients with celiac disease: A cross-sectional observational study. *Andrology* **2022**, *10*, 910–918. [CrossRef] [PubMed]
54. Santonicola, A.; Iovino, P.; Cappello, C.; Capone, P.; Andreozzi, P.; Ciacci, C. From menarche to menopause: The fertile life span of celiac women. *Menopause* **2011**, *18*, 1125–1130. [CrossRef]
55. Nenna, R.; Mennini, M.; Petrarca, L.; Bonamico, M. Immediate effect on fertility of a gluten-free diet in women with untreated coeliac disease. *Gut* **2011**, *60*, 1023–1024. [CrossRef]
56. Alecsandru, D.; López-Palacios, N.; Castaño, M.; Aparicio, P.; García-Velasco, J.A.; Núñez, C. Exploring undiagnosed celiac disease in women with recurrent reproductive failure: The gluten-free diet could improve reproductive outcomes. *Am. J. Reprod. Immunol.* **2020**, *83*, e13209. [CrossRef]
57. Ayoub, A.; Firwana, M.; Amjahdi, A.; Rahaoui, A.; Benelbarhdadi, I.; Zahra, A.F. Evolution of Reproductive Disorders Related to Celiac Disease under Gluten-free Diet. *Int. J. Celiac Dis.* **2017**, *5*, 69–71. [CrossRef]
58. Lebwohl, B.; Rubio-Tapia, A.; Assiri, A.; Newland, C.; Guandalini, S. Diagnosis of celiac disease. *Gastrointest. Endosc. Clin. N. Am.* **2012**, *22*, 661–677. [CrossRef]
59. Ciacci, C.; Santonicola, A. Editorial: Coeliac Disease and Women's Reproductive Health: A Lifelong Challenge. *Aliment. Pharmacol. Ther.* **2025**, *61*, 1703–1704. [CrossRef]
60. Grode, L.; Møller Jensen, T.; Parkner, T.; Agerholm, I.E.; Humaidan, P.; Hammer Bech, B.; Ramlau-Hansen, C. Diagnostic Accuracy of a Point-of-Care Test for Celiac Disease Antibody Screening among Infertile Patients. *Inflamm. Intest. Dis.* **2019**, *4*, 123–130. [CrossRef]
61. Krawczyk, A.; Kretek, A.; Pluta, D.; Kowalczyk, K.; Czech, I.; Radosz, P.; Madej, P. Gluten-free diet—Remedy for infertility or dangerous trend? *Ginekol. Pol.* **2022**, *93*, 422–426. [CrossRef] [PubMed]

nutrients

MDPI

Article

Coeliac Disease Case–Control Study: Has the Time Come to Explore beyond Patients at Risk?

Gemma Castillejo [1,*], Carlos Ochoa-Sangrador [2], David Pérez-Solís [3], Maria Luz Cilleruelo [4], Ester Donat [5], Jose Ignacio García-Burriel [6], Félix Sánchez-Valverde [7], Salvador Garcia-Calatayud [8], Francisco Javier Eizaguirre [9], Eva Martinez-Ojinaga [10], Patricia Barros [11], Rosaura Leis [12], Jose Carlos Salazar [13], Josefa Barrio [14], Luis Peña-Quintana [15], Verónica Luque [16], Isabel Polanco [10], Carmen Ribes [5] and Enriqueta Roman [4] on behalf of the Coeliac Disease Working Group of the Spanish Paediatric Gastroenterology, Hepatology and Nutrition Society (SEGHNP)

1 Unitat de Recerca en Pediatria, Hospital Universitari Sant Joan de Reus, Nutrició i Desenvolupament Humà, IISPV, Universitat Rovira i Virgili, 43204 Reus, Spain
2 Complejo Asistencial de Zamora, 49022 Zamora, Spain
3 Pediatrics, Hospital Universitario San Agustín, 33401 Avilés, Spain
4 Hospital Universitario Puerta de Hierro, Majadahonda, 28222 Madrid, Spain
5 Pediatric Gastroenterology and Hepatology Unit, Celiac Disease and Digestive Immunopathology Unit, Instituto de Investigación Sanitaria La Fe, Hospital Universitari i Politècnic La Fe, 46026 Valencia, Spain
6 Complejo Hospitalario Universitario de Vigo, 36312 Vigo, Spain
7 Navarre Children's Nutrition and Digestive Study Group (GENDINA), Department of Paediatrics, NAVARRA BIOMED, University Hospital of Navarra, 31008 Pamplona, Spain
8 Hospital Universitario Marques de Valdecilla, 39008 Santander, Spain
9 Paediatric Gastroenterology, Hepatology and Nutrition Unit, Hospital Universitario Donostia, 20006 San Sebastian, Spain
10 Department of Pediatric Gastroenterology, Hospital Universitario La Paz, 28046 Madrid, Spain
11 Hospital San Pedro de Alcántara, 10071 Cáceres, Spain
12 Unit of Pediatrics Gastroenterology, Hepatology and Nutrition, Pediatrics Department, Hospital Clínico Universitario de Santiago-USC, IDIS, CiberObn, 15706 Santiago de Compostela, Spain
13 Hospital Universitario Infantil Virgen del Rocío, 41013 Sevilla, Spain
14 Hospital Universitario de Fuenlabrada, Fuenlabrada, 28942 Madrid, Spain
15 Pediatric Gastroenterology, Hepatology and Nutrition Unit, Complejo Hospitalario Universitario Insular Materno-Infantil, CIBEROBN ISCIII-Universidad de Las Palmas de Gran Canaria, 35016 Gran Canaria, Spain
16 Unitat de Recerca en Pediatria, Nutrició i Desenvolupament Humà, Universitat Rovira i Virgili, 43007 Tarragona, Spain
* Correspondence: gemma.castillejo@urv.cat

Abstract: The worldwide prevalence of asymptomatic coeliac disease (CD) is increasing, which is in part due to the routine screening of children with risk factors. Both symptomatic and asymptomatic patients with CD are at risk of long-term complications. The objective of this study was to compare the clinical characteristics of asymptomatic and symptomatic children at the time of CD diagnosis. A case–control study was conducted using data from a cohort of 4838 CD patients recruited from 73 centers across Spain between 2011 and 2017. A total of 468 asymptomatic patients (cases) were selected and matched by age and sex with 468 symptomatic patients (controls). Clinical data, including any reported symptoms, as well as serologic, genetic, and histopathologic data were collected. No significant differences were found between the two groups in most clinical variables, nor in the degree of intestinal lesion. However, the asymptomatic patients were taller (height z-score −0.12 (1.06) vs. −0.45 (1.19), $p < 0.001$) and were less likely to have anti transglutaminase IgA antibodies ≥ 10 times the upper normal limit (66.2% vs. 758.4%, $p = 0.002$). Among the 37.1% of asymptomatic patients who were not screened for CD due to the absence of risk factors, only 34% were truly asymptomatic, while the remaining 66% reported non-specific CD-related symptoms. Therefore, expanding CD screening to any child who undergoes a blood test could reduce the burden of care for some children, as many of those considered asymptomatic reported non-specific CD-related symptoms.

Keywords: coeliac disease; pediatric gastroenterology; screening; general practice

1. Introduction

Coeliac disease (CD) is an immune-mediated systemic disorder triggered by gluten and related prolamins in genetically susceptible individuals. It is characterized by a variable combination of gluten-dependent clinical manifestations, CD-specific antibodies, HLA-DQ2/8 haplotypes, and enteropathy [1]. Over the past few decades, the presentation of CD has changed worldwide, with the diagnosis occurring at an older age [2] and a greater number of patients being diagnosed with more subtle symptoms or even as asymptomatic [3]. This change is partly due to the recognition that the disease can occur at any age and the introduction of screening in high-risk children, who are often asymptomatic. Moreover, the asymptomatic CD is becoming more common, as shown by some studies in which almost 1% of asymptomatic healthy adolescents screened (without risk factors for CD) had CD [4]. Screening is recommended for first-degree relatives of CD patients and in children with a concomitant disease (chromosomal abnormalities such as Downs, Turner, or Williams syndrome, as well as patients with another autoimmune disease, such as type 1 diabetes, autoimmune thyroid, or autoimmune hepatitis, among others), as CD patients have a 3- to 10-fold higher risk of developing another autoimmune disease [5–8]. It is worth noting that a recent US mass screening study performed in 9973 children found that 90% of asymptomatic positive children did not have a first-degree relative affected with CD [9]. This highlights the importance of widespread screening for CD, as relying solely on symptoms or risk factors such as family history may miss many cases. Furthermore, it is important to note that other studies have found that the serological, histological, and genetic characteristics of symptomatic and asymptomatic CD patients are similar [10,11]. Given the high prevalence of this disease [12], particularly in Europe, and the potential for serious complications if left untreated [13], it is crucial to investigate the characteristics of patients with or without symptoms at the time of diagnosis. This information can be used to inform decision-making in the healthcare practice. The aim of this study is to compare the characteristics of asymptomatic and symptomatic CD patients at the time of diagnosis.

2. Materials and Methods

2.1. Study Design and Population

The present study was designed as a case–control study, embedded in the REPAC2 cohort [14]. This was a nationwide, prospective, observational, multicenter registry of new CD cases recorded between January 2011 and June 2017. The CD Working Group of the Spanish Gastroenterology, Hepatology, and Pediatric Nutrition Society (SEGHNP) invited all pediatric gastroenterology departments in Spain to participate in the study. Of the 117 pediatric gastroenterology units in Spain, 73 (62.4%) from 15 of the 17 Spanish regions agreed to participate. The inclusion criteria for this study were patients under 15 years of age who were diagnosed with CD at participating centers after the study start date. To be included in the cohort, patients had to meet the diagnostic criteria established by the European Society for Pediatric Gastroenterology Hepatology and Nutrition (ESPGHAN) at the time of diagnosis. For patients diagnosed before 2011, the 1990 ESPGHAN criteria were used [15], while for those diagnosed since 2011, the 2012 criteria were used [16]. To clarify, before 2011, all patients diagnosed with CD had to undergo an intestinal biopsy for diagnosis. However, since 2012, patients can be diagnosed without undergoing an intestinal biopsy, if they meet the diagnostic criteria established by the ESPGHAN. Asymptomatic CD cases and a group of symptomatic controls were selected for the study, with each case being matched 1:1 by center, age, and sex. Children were considered asymptomatic if they did not have any CD-suggestive symptoms according to the ESPGHAN diagnostic guidelines [1,16]. However, some of the so-called asymptomatic children had other complaints that were not considered in the guidelines and were thus categorized as having "non-specific CD symptoms" for the purposes of the study.

2.2. Data Analysis and Management

The data for this study were collected through an electronic questionnaire hosted on the SEGHNP website. The questionnaire collected information on various aspects of the patient's medical history, including demographics, mode of delivery, breastfeeding history, CD family history, CD-specific symptoms, height and weight, associated conditions, serology, biopsy, and genetic results. Clinical presentations were classified as either asymptomatic or symptomatic based on the presence or absence of symptoms established by the ESPGHAN diagnostic guidelines [1,16]. Symptomatic children had at least one of the signs or symptoms mentioned in the guidelines: chronic or intermittent abdominal pain, diarrhea, constipation or bloating, distended abdomen, recurrent nausea and/or vomiting, tiredness and lethargy, weight loss, failure-to-thrive, stunted growth/short stature, delayed puberty, amenorrhea, irritability, chronic fatigue, neuropathy, arthritis/arthralgia, chronic iron-deficiency anemia, decreased bone mineralization, recurrent aphthous stomatitis, dermatitis herpetiformis, dental enamel defects, and abnormal liver biochemistry. Asymptomatic patients were evaluated to determine if they belonged to a risk group, such as first-degree relatives of patients with celiac disease, those who already had another autoimmune disease, and those with chromosomal diseases, to see if a blood test for CD detection was indicated. The study team collected information on why the blood test was performed for asymptomatic patients who did not belong to a high-risk group. The responses were collected in an open text box and analyzed to determine the reason for the blood test. If data were missing, patients were not excluded, and no imputation was performed. To summarize, asymptomatic patients were classified into three groups: the first group included patients with high-risk factors such as first-degree relatives of CD, and those with other autoimmune or chromosomal diseases. The second group included asymptomatic children who had symptoms not listed in the guidelines (non-specific CD symptoms), and the third group included patients with no symptoms at all.

To calculate the z-scores for height, weight, and body mass index (BMI), the study used the growth references and standards provided by the World Health Organization (WHO) [17,18]. A z-score of 0 indicates that a child's measurement is equal to the median, while a z-score of +1 or −1 indicates that the measurement is one standard deviation above or below the median, respectively.

Serology tests for celiac disease were performed at each participating center to detect anti transglutaminase IgA antibodies (TGA-IgA) and anti endomysial IgA antibodies (EMA-IgA) based on the available methods in their laboratories, with specific cut-off values determined for each method. The antibody titer for each patient was recorded, along with the cut-off value used. HLA typing was also performed locally, and patients were grouped as DQ2 or DQ8 based on the results. Some centers performed complete genotyping, while others determined only DQ2/8 positivity or negativity. All patients underwent fibrogastroduodenoscopy, which was performed under sedation, and macroscopic and microscopic findings were recorded. The biopsy samples were evaluated by the pathologist at each center and classified according to the Marsh–Oberhuber classification. [19]. In this study, samples classified as Marsh 2 to 3 according to the Marsh–Oberhuber classification were considered indicative of CD [16].

2.3. Statistical Analysis

The study was designed with an expected sample size of 468 cases and 468 controls, with a power of 86.8% and an alpha error of 0.05 to estimate differences of more than 10% between groups. The distribution of continuous variables was assessed using histograms and Kolmogorov–Smirnov test. Continuous variables were reported as mean and standard deviation or median and interquartile range (IQR) based on their distribution. Chi-squared tests were used for group comparisons for categorical variables, while Student's *t*-test and

ANOVA or Mann–Whitney U-tests and Kruskal–Wallis test were used for group comparisons for continuous variables, depending on their distribution. Statistical significance was accepted at $p < 0.05$, and IBM SPSS Statistics version 26 (IBM Corp., Armonk, NY, USA) was used for all statistical analyses.

2.4. Ethics and Approvals

The investigations were carried out according to the principles of the Declaration of Helsinki. Informed consent was obtained from the parents or legal guardians of the participants. This study was approved by the Research Ethics Committee of the Hospital Universitario Puerta de Hierro, Majadahonda, Madrid (263.2011), and individually, by all participating centers.

3. Results

The study included a total of 4838 celiac children, and out of these, 468 were identified as asymptomatic (9.67% of the total population). The mean age of the asymptomatic patients was 7.8 years, with an interquartile range of 4.7–11.2 years. These 468 asymptomatic coeliac patients (cases) were then matched with 468 symptomatic coeliac patients to serve as controls for the study.

During randomization, we selected 97 non-biopsy controls who were diagnosed after 2012 and met the criteria for using that approach. Since we were unsure whether there were differences between asymptomatic and symptomatic patients depending on whether they underwent a biopsy, we performed duplicate analyses. One set of the analyses included the controls randomly selected, which included 97 cases without a biopsy, while the other set only selected the controls who were diagnosed with a biopsy. However, no significant differences were found between the two analyses. Therefore, we used the randomly selected cases for the analyses, and the 97 children diagnosed without a biopsy have missing values of the Marsh lesion grade.

Table 1 shows the comparative characteristics in cases and controls.

Table 1. Characteristics of asymptomatic and symptomatic patients at diagnosis.

	Cases (n = 468) Asymptomatic at Diagnosis	**Controls (n = 468) Symptomatic at Diagnosis**	***p*-Value**
Background information			
Male sex	199 (42.5%)	199 (42.5%)	NS
Age (years)	8.2 (5.3–11.4)	7.8 (4.8–11.2)	NS
Delivery type (C section)	87 (18.6)	107 (22.9)	NS
Breastfeeding	103 (76.3)	87 (79.2)	NS
Rotavirus vaccination	69 (14.7)	73 (15.6)	NS
Age at gluten introduction (months)	6 (6–8)	6.5 (6–8)	NS
Weight (z-score)	0.16 (1.06)	−0.45 (1.19)	<0.001
Height (z-score)	−0.12 (1.06)	−0.54 (1.22)	<0.001
BMI (z-score)	0.32 (1.15)	−0.19 (1.19)	<0.001
Risk factors			
Relatives with CD			<0.001
No	250 (54.1%)	383 (82.7%)	
First degree	161 (34.8%)	29 (6.3%)	
Second degree	42 (9.1%)	47 (10.2%)	
First and second degree	9 (1.9%)	4 (0.9%)	
Diabetes	62 (13.4%)	4 (0.9%)	<0.001
Thyroiditis	18 (3.9%)	5 (1.1%)	0.006
Down Syndrome	10 (2.2%)	0 (0.0%)	0.001
Laboratory parameters			
IgA antiendomysium +	325 (97.3) [a]	328 (98.2) [a]	NS
TGA-IgA ≥ 10xUNL	310 (66.2)	353 (75.4)	0.002
HLA	(n = 409)	(n = 393)	NS
DQ2	345 (84.4%)	338 (86.0%)	

Table 1. *Cont.*

	Cases (n = 468) Asymptomatic at Diagnosis	Controls (n = 468) Symptomatic at Diagnosis	p-Value
DQ2/DQ8	40 (9.8%)	34 (8.7%)	
DQ8	20 (4.9%)	11 (2.8%)	
Others	4 (1.0%)	10 (2.5%)	
Marsh lesion grade	(n = 468)	(n = 371)	0.017 [b]
2	29 (6.2%)	17 (4.6%)	
3a	162 (34.6%)	96 (25.9%)	0.002 [c]
3b	188 (40.2%)	181 (48.8%)	
3c	89 (19.0%)	77 (20.8%)	

N (%) or mean (SD) or median (interquartile range). [a] Only available in 334. [b] Chi2 linear trend. [c] Post hoc analysis. Marsh 2 or 3a versus 3b or 3c. BMI: body mass index; CD: coeliac disease; UNL: upper normal limit; and TGA: anti transglutaminase IgA antibodies.

No significant differences were found between the two groups in terms of mode of delivery, breastfeeding, rotavirus vaccination, age at gluten introduction, anti endomysial IgA antibody positivity, or HLA type. The asymptomatic group exhibited a higher prevalence of risk factors, including autoimmune diseases such as type 1 diabetes mellitus and thyroiditis, Downs syndrome, and a first-degree family member with celiac disease compared to the symptomatic group. Moreover, asymptomatic children had slightly higher weight and height measurements than the symptomatic children (Figure 1).

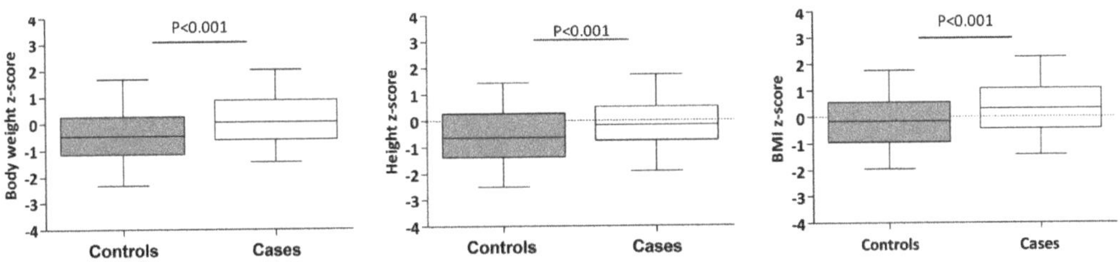

Figure 1. Anthropometrical measurements of cases and controls at diagnosis.

Notably, the height of symptomatic children was below the mean for the general population, while in the asymptomatic cases, it was distributed around the normal values of the population.

Compared to symptomatic patients, asymptomatic patients were less likely to have a TGA-IgA value $\geq$ 10 times the upper limit of normal (ULN) (66% vs. 75%, p = 0.002) and had a higher proportion of milder lesions (Marsh 2 and 3a), while the symptomatic controls had a greater proportion of Marsh 3b and 3c. A review of the reasons behind conducting TGA-IgA tests on asymptomatic patients demonstrated that a significant proportion (up to 61.1%) of them belonged to high-risk groups identified by the ESPGHAN diagnostic protocol, such as individuals with genetic syndromes, first-degree relatives of CD patients, or other autoimmune diseases. However, 37.1% of the tests were performed without following the protocol, with some patients exhibiting non-specific symptoms associated with CD (24.5%), while others were completely asymptomatic (12.6%) (Figure 2).

Upon further investigation, recruiters reached out to families to inquire about the reason for conducting TGA-IgA tests on asymptomatic children. Of the 37.1% of patients without risk factors, 12.6% underwent testing as part of non-urgent preoperative checks, evaluations for familial hypercholesterolemia, or routine assessments upon starting care with a new pediatrician or family doctor. The remaining 24.5% had a medical concern unrelated to CD, such as allergy evaluations for recurring wheezing, food or respiratory allergies, atopic dermatitis, or urticaria, as well as assessments for non-specific skin lesions such as eczema or lichen, chest pain, halitosis, dizziness, recurrent URTIs, polyphagia, syncope, or dysphagia.

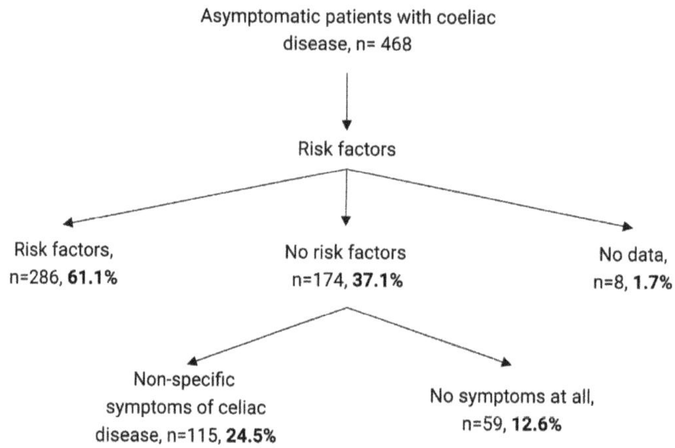

Figure 2. Categorization of cases.

Table 2 shows the characteristics of all asymptomatic cases according to the reason for screening.

Table 2. Asymptomatic cases according to the reason for screening *.

	CD Risk Factors [a] *n* = 286	**Non-Specific CD Symptoms** [b] *n* = 115	**Other Reasons** *n* = 59	*p*-**Value**
Background information				
Male sex (% from total)	126 (44.1%)	45 (39.1%)	23 (39.0%)	0.577
Age (years)	8.3 (5.3–11.4)	8.1 (4.7–11.2)	7.6 (4.4–11.5)	0.603
Age at gluten introduction (months)	7 (6–8)	6 (6–7)	6 (6–7)	0.022
Weight (z-score)	0.15 (0.97)	0.14 (1.30)	0.12 (0.88)	0.973
Height (z-score)	−0.16 (1.02)	−0.07 (1.21)	−0.16 (0.89)	0.716
BMI (z-score)	0.35 (1.03)	0.24 (1.41)	0.29 (1.15)	0.686
Laboratory parameters	*n* (% from total)			
IgA antiendomysium +	196 (96.5%)	91 (98.9%)	30 (96.7%)	0.511
TGA-IgA ≥ 10xUNL	192 (67.1%)	74 (64.3%)	40 (67.8%)	0.550
HLA				NS
DQ2	205 (82.3%)	85 (84.2%)	48 (92.3%)	
DQ2/DQ8	29 (11.6%)	8 (7.9%)	3 (5.8%)	
DQ8	12 (4.8%)	7 (6.9%)	1 (1.9%)	
Others	3 (1.2%)	1 (1.0%)	0 (0.0%)	
Marsh lesion grade				NS
2	13 (4.5%)	11 (9.6%)	5 (8.5%)	
3a	108 (37.8%)	31 (27.0%)	19 (32.2%)	
3b	104 (36.4%)	50 (43.5%)	31 (52.5%)	
3c	61 (21.3%)	23 (20.0%)	4 (6.8%)	

* For 8 patients, no reason for screening was noted in the open box text N (%) or mean (SD) or median (interquartile range). [a] Family history of CD: 186, endocrine diseases: 82 (diabetes and hypothyroidism), genetic disorders: 12 (Downs syndrome; Williams syndrome), and rheumatic diseases: 6 (juvenile idiopathic arthritis) [b] Non-specific CD symptoms, such as allergy studies, non-specific skin lesions, halitosis, dizziness, and recurrent URIs, among others.

Among the asymptomatic cases, the only significant difference found was related to the age of gluten introduction, with those with a family history of CD introducing gluten at a later age compared to those without such a history (months; $p = 0.022$). No other significant differences were found.

4. Discussion

To the best of our knowledge, this case–control study represents the largest sample of asymptomatic coeliac patients that have been characterized to date. The findings in this study suggest that the diagnosis of CD in asymptomatic patients is not limited to high-risk groups, and this detailed analysis indicates that asymptomatic CD patients, regardless of their risk group status, share similar characteristics. The study revealed that although celiac disease may present as milder in asymptomatic cases (with lower TGA-IgA levels and less severe intestinal damage), these variations do not have any significant impact on the diagnosis. As we have seen in the results of this study, families with celiac relatives may delay introducing gluten to their children's diets due to concerns about the potential risk of developing celiac disease. Further, it has been described that undiagnosed CD can have significant impacts on one's physical and general development, leading to long-term complications [10,20], such as anemia, dental enamel defects [21], osteoporosis [22,23], or underachievement [24,25], which can remain permanent if CD is not treated [13].

The observations of the CD patients in the studied population align with previous research findings, indicating that height impairment in children can occur before the onset of symptoms [26,27]. The potential for irreversible growth impairment in the pediatric age group makes early detection and treatment of CD crucial. It has been described that almost half of the asymptomatic patients have minor symptoms that may go unnoticed until they improve after initiating the gluten-free diet (GFD) [10,28–30]. A Dutch study conducted some years ago proposed that patients be given the option to decide for themselves whether to adhere to a GFD, as some asymptomatic individuals who initially declined the diet may choose to begin it early if symptoms eventually worsen [29].

The proportion of asymptomatic patients in the studied population was 9.67%, which is consistent with other international cohorts such as those from Finland [10], the UK [31], Saudi Arabia [32], the Netherlands [33], and New Zealand [34]. However, a central European cohort showed a higher percentage of asymptomatic cases, ranging from 12.1% in Croatia to 26.5% in Italy [35]. The reason for specifically studying asymptomatic patients in this cohort is due to the increasing worldwide prevalence of asymptomatic cases, as mentioned earlier [3]. An indication of the increasing importance of this group of asymptomatic patients is reflected in the fact that, for the first time, the revised ESPGHAN criteria published in 2020 allow for diagnosis without biopsy in asymptomatic patients, the majority of whom belong to high-risk groups, as was significantly observed in this cohort. However, as results from this study and others [9] have shown, it may not be sufficient to limit CD screening to at-risk groups. In the present study, over a third of asymptomatic children were diagnosed due to TGA-IgA being included as a basic parameter in blood tests, even though this is not indicated by diagnosis guidelines. While this determination is justified in asymptomatic patients from risk groups due to the increase in prevalence, we have observed that the other two groups of asymptomatic patients behave the same. This leads the authors to question whether the inclusion of TGA-IgA plus total IgA as part of the basic biochemical profile may be justified in children whose pediatrician or family practitioner decides to carry out a blood test. This approach could reduce the gap between diagnosed and undiagnosed patients in both children and adults, which the literature has placed at between 75 and 90% over the years [26,36–38]. Bringing the diagnosis forward to the pediatric age could also help avoid the overuse of healthcare services and medication that have been described prior to CD diagnosis in both pediatric and adult age groups [39–43], as well as the delay in diagnosis in adulthood, which has been reported to be up to 10 years [44], despite the presence of CD-suggestive symptoms. The authors would like to emphasize that while CD screening is mandatory in at-risk children and meets most of the screening criteria set by the World Health Organization, universal screening for the general population, at least in adults, is currently controversial [45], although it seems to be cost-effective [43,46]. In the meantime, an opportunistic approach to CD screening could be considered for non-at-risk children who undergo blood testing for unrelated conditions. Furthermore, other recent studies have also suggested broader screening beyond just at-risk groups [9,47]. Blood testing is not common in pediatric practice and is usually performed for health or developmental reasons.

However, two important points should be emphasized. First, our study found that asymptomatic patients are less likely to have TGA-IgA levels above 10 times the UNL, which implies that they are more likely to require a biopsy to confirm the diagnosis. Second, some patients with potential CD are asymptomatic, and therefore, transient low positive serology results may be found [48]. Therefore, CD diagnosis in children, especially those with low–intermediate TGA values, should be performed in centers with sufficient experience and a carefully validated laboratory method using appropriate tests. If a child's blood test in a general pediatric practice shows a TGA-IgA level above the threshold, the child should be referred to a specialized center for a definitive diagnosis before starting a GFD, since the misdiagnosis of CD can have long-lasting consequences. Up to 55% of children with potential CD may never develop overt CD [49–52].

The authors have identified some reasons for not performing TGA-IgA testing in asymptomatic individuals who are not part of high-risk populations. One reason may be the assumption that these patients would have lower compliance with the GFD and that asymptomatic individuals would not benefit from the GFD. However, little evidence suggests otherwise [28], and in general, compliance with a GFD among asymptomatic CD patients is generally good, particularly in children [28,53]. In some cases, compliance can be worse, as has been observed in a small group of patients [54]. In addition, the assumption that asymptomatic individuals would not benefit from the GFD may not be entirely accurate. Only 12.8% of the patients in this cohort were truly asymptomatic (Figure 2), and other studies have reported similar results, with many asymptomatic patients presenting with minor symptoms that improve after starting the GFD [10,28,30]. Concerns about the potential negative impact of starting a lifelong GFD without symptoms may also be unfounded. Recent studies comparing the quality of life and dietary adherence of children diagnosed through screening or symptoms have shown no difference between the two groups [29,53]. Instead, some authors suggest a different approach to the treatment and follow-up of this patient group to avoid decreased quality of life or increased anxiety [55]. Allowing patients to make their own decision may also be appropriate, as some initially asymptomatic patients who declined the diet may later choose to start it as their symptoms worsen [29].

Based on the mean prevalence of 0.74% [56] for undiagnosed CD/asymptomatic patients (with a range of 0.10–3.03%), including TGA-IgA as part of the basic analysis profile in children undergoing blood testing can allow the diagnosis of up to 280/100,000 children without risk factors, considering that 37.1% of the asymptomatic children in the authors' study were diagnosed with CD. Therefore, the proposed "diagnostic approach of opportunity" could be more cost-effective than screening the general population.

Additional studies are needed to evaluate the actual cost-effectiveness of this approach, its generalizability, and whether follow-up for these patients should be designed differently to identify any issues arising from adherence to a strict diet.

5. Conclusions

Currently, there are still many undiagnosed CD patients. Screening has been implemented in children belonging to risk groups for CD, such as first-degree relatives or those affected by another autoimmune or chromosomal disease. Asymptomatic cases are usually diagnosed in these at-risk populations. This study's findings have allowed for the verification of symptomatic and asymptomatic patients being identical in a large cohort; the only difference is that the asymptomatic patients present less severe intestinal damage and less impact on their nutritional state, which is beneficial in the pediatric age since they are in a period of growth.

Considering the fact that other studies have shown that complications are possible even in asymptomatic patients, but universal screening in the general population remains controversial, we propose an opportunistic screening approach beyond children at risk of CD. Therefore, we suggest exploring the existence of CD in non-at-risk children who undergo a blood test for an unrelated condition. Blood testing is not that common in pediatric practice, and when it is performed, it is usually for health or developmental reasons. By adopting this opportunistic approach, the burden of care and the risk of possible long-term complications in asymptomatic cases would be reduced. Further studies are needed to determine the cost-effectiveness of this approach and whether follow-up care should be designed differently to identify problems arising from adherence to a strict diet.

Supplementary Materials: The following supporting information can be downloaded at: https://www.mdpi.com/article/10.3390/nu15051267/s1. File S1: Complete list of authors.

Author Contributions: Conceptualization G.C., C.O.-S., D.P.-S., M.L.C., E.D. and E.R.; investigation: all authors except V.L.; methodology, G.C. and C.O.-S.; software, D.P.-S., E.R. and M.L.C.; validation, G.C., C.O.-S. and V.L.; formal analysis, C.O.-S., V.L. and D.P.-S.; data curation, D.P.-S. and G.C.; writing—original draft preparation, G.C.; writing—review and editing, G.C., C.O.-S., D.P.-S., M.L.C., E.D., J.I.G.-B., F.S.-V., S.G.-C., F.J.E., E.M.-O., P.B., R.L., J.C.S., J.B., L.P.-Q., V.L., I.P., C.R. and E.R.; supervision, E.R. All authors have read and agreed to the published version of the manuscript.

Funding: This research received no external funding.

Institutional Review Board Statement: The study was conducted in accordance with the Declaration of Helsinki and was approved by the Research Ethics Committee of the Hospital Universitario Puerta de Hierro, Majadahonda, Madrid (263.2011), and individually, by all participating centers.

Informed Consent Statement: Informed consent was obtained from all subjects involved in the study.

Data Availability Statement: Data are available on request.

Acknowledgments: The authors would like to thank all the members of the SEGHNP CD Working Group, who participated as recruiters, for their invaluable contributions to this project. They are listed as collaborators in the Supplemental Materials. Additionally, Rosa Mª Quintero, for her help in translation.

Conflicts of Interest: The authors declare no conflict of interest.

References

1. Husby, S.; Koletzko, S.; Korponay-Szabó, I.; Kurppa, K.; Mearin, M.L.; Ribes-Koninckx, C.; Wessels, M. European Society Paediatric Gastroenterology, Hepatology and Nutrition Guidelines for Diagnosing Coeliac Disease 2020. *J. Pediatr. Gastroenterol. Nutr.* **2020**, *70*, 141–156. [CrossRef]
2. Mäki, M.; Kallonen, K.; Lähdeaho, M.L.; Visakorpi, J.K. Changing Pattern of Childhood Coeliac Disease in Finland. *Acta Pediatr. Scand.* **1988**, *77*, 408–412. [CrossRef]
3. Popp, A.; Mäki, M. Changing pattern of childhood celiac disease epidemiology: Contributing factors. *Front. Pediatr.* **2019**, *7*, 357. [CrossRef] [PubMed]
4. Rutz, R.; Ritzler, E.; Fierz, W.; Herzog, D. Prevalence of asymptomatic celiac disease in adolescents of eastern Switzerland. *Swiss Med. Wkly.* **2002**, *132*, 43–47. [CrossRef] [PubMed]
5. Bibbò, S.; Pes, G.M.; Usai-Satta, P.; Salis, R.; Soro, S.; Colosso, B.M.Q.; Dore, M.P. Chronic autoimmune disorders are increased in coeliac disease. *Medicine* **2017**, *96*, e8562. [CrossRef]
6. Neuhausen, S.L.; Steele, L.; Ryan, S.; Mousavi, M.; Pinto, M.; Osann, K.E.; Zone, J.J. Co-occurrence of celiac disease and other autoimmune diseases in celiacs and their first-degree relatives. *J. Autoimmun.* **2008**, *31*, 160–165. [CrossRef] [PubMed]
7. Emilsson, L.; Wijmenga, C.; Murray, J.A.; Ludvigsson, J.F. Autoimmune Disease in First-Degree Relatives and Spouses of Individuals with Celiac Disease. *Clin. Gastroenterol. Hepatol.* **2015**, *13*, 1271–1277. [CrossRef]
8. Kahaly, G.; Frommer, L.; Schuppan, D. Celiac Disease and Glandular Autoimmunity. *Nutrients* **2018**, *10*, 814. [CrossRef]
9. Stahl, M.G.; Geno Rasmussen, C.; Dong, F.; Waugh, K.; Norris, J.M.; Baxter, J.; ASK Study Group. Mass Screening for Celiac Disease: The Autoimmunity Screening for Kids Study. *Am. J. Gastroenterol.* **2021**, *116*, 180–187. [CrossRef]
10. Kivelä, L.; Kaukinen, K.; Huhtala, H.; Lähdeaho, M.L.; Mäki, M.; Kurppa, K. At-Risk Screened Children with Celiac Disease are Comparable in Disease Severity and Dietary Adherence to Those Found because of Clinical Suspicion: A Large Cohort Study. *J. Pediatr.* **2017**, *183*, 115–121. [CrossRef]
11. Paul, S.P.; Sandhu, B.K.; Spray, C.H.; Basude, D.; Ramani, P. Evidence Supporting Serology-based Pathway for Diagnosing Celiac Disease in Asymptomatic Children from High-risk Groups. *J. Pediatr. Gastroenterol. Nutr.* **2018**, *66*, 641–644. [CrossRef] [PubMed]
12. Catassi, C.; Verdu, E.F.; Bai, J.C.; Lionetti, E. Coeliac disease. *Lancet* **2022**, *399*, 2413–2426. [CrossRef] [PubMed]

13. Laurikka, P.; Kivelä, L.; Kurppa, K.; Kaukinen, K. Review article: Systemic consequences of coeliac disease. *Aliment. Pharmacol. Ther.* **2022**, *56* (Suppl. S1), S64–S72. [CrossRef]
14. Solís, D.P.; Pascual, M.L.C.; Sangrador, C.O.; Burriel, J.I.G.; Visus, F.S.V.; Arocena, F.J.E.; Riechmann, E.R. Spanish National Registry of Paediatric Coeliac Disease: Changes in the Clinical Presentation in the 21st Century. *J. Pediatr. Gastroenterol. Nutr.* **2022**, *74*, 805–811. [CrossRef] [PubMed]
15. Walker-Smith, J.A. Revised criteria for diagnosis of coeliac disease Report of Working Group of European Society of Paediatric Gastroenterology and Nutrition. *Arch. Dis. Child.* **1990**, *65*, 909–911.
16. Husby, S.; Koletzko, S.; Korponay-Szabó, I.R.; Mearin, M.L.; Phillips, A.; Shamir, R.; ESPGHAN Gastroenterology Committee. European society for pediatric gastroenterology, hepatology, and nutrition guidelines for the diagnosis of coeliac disease. *J. Pediatr. Gastroenterol. Nutr.* **2012**, *54*, 136–160. [CrossRef]
17. WHO Multicentre Growth Reference Study Group. WHO Child Growth Standards based on length/height, weight and age. *Acta Paediatr. Suppl.* **2006**, *450*, 76–85.
18. De Onis, M. Development of a WHO growth reference for school-aged children and adolescents. *Bull. World Health Organ.* **2007**, *85*, 660–667. [CrossRef] [PubMed]
19. Oberhuber, G.; Granditsch, G.; Vogelsang, H. The histopathology of coeliac disease: Time for a standardized report scheme for pathologists. *Eur. J. Gastroenterol. Hepatol.* **1999**, *11*, 1185–1194. [CrossRef]
20. Bonamico, M.; Nenna, R. Implications of mass screening for childhood celiac disease. *Ped. Health* **2009**, *3*, 413–415. [CrossRef]
21. Krzywicka, B.; Herman, K.; Kowalczyk-Zając, M.; Pytrus, T. Celiac Disease and Its Impact on the Oral Health Status—Review of the Literature. *Adv. Clin. Exp. Med.* **2014**, *23*, 675–681. [CrossRef] [PubMed]
22. Turner, J.; Pellerin, G.; Mager, D. Prevalence of Metabolic Bone Disease in Children with Celiac Disease Is Independent of Symptoms at Diagnosis. *J. Pediatr. Gastroenterol. Nutr.* **2009**, *49*, 589–593. [CrossRef]
23. Björck, S.; Brundin, C.; Karlsson, M.; Agardh, D. Reduced Bone Mineral Density in Children with Screening-detected Celiac Disease. *J. Pediatr. Gastroenterol. Nutr.* **2017**, *65*, 526–532. [CrossRef]
24. Verkasalo, M.A.; Raitakari, O.T.; Viikari, J.; Marniemi, J.; Savilahti, E. Undiagnosed silent coeliac disease: A risk for underachievement? *Scand. J. Gastroenterol.* **2005**, *40*, 1407–1412. [CrossRef]
25. Nurminen, S.; Kivelä, L.; Taavela, J.; Huhtala, H.; Mäki, M.; Kaukinen, K.; Kurppa, K. Factors associated with growth disturbance at celiac disease diagnosis in children: A retrospective cohort study. *BMC Gastroenterol.* **2015**, *15*, 125. [CrossRef]
26. Bingley, P.J.; Norcross, A.J.; Lock, R.J.; Ness, A.R.; Jones, R.W. Undiagnosed coeliac disease at age seven: Population based prospective birth cohort study. *BMJ* **2004**, *328*, 322–323. [CrossRef]
27. Auricchio, R.; Stellato, P.; Bruzzese, D.; Cielo, D.; Chiurazzi, A.; Galatola, M.; Greco, L. Growth rate of coeliac children is compromised before the onset of the disease. *Arch. Dis. Child.* **2020**, *105*, 964–968. [CrossRef] [PubMed]
28. Kivelä, L.; Popp, A.; Arvola, T.; Huhtala, H.; Kaukinen, K.; Kurppa, K. Long-term health and treatment outcomes in adult coeliac disease patients diagnosed by screening in childhood. *United Eur. Gastroenterol. J.* **2018**, *6*, 1022–1031. [CrossRef] [PubMed]
29. Van Koppen, E.J.; Schweizer, J.J.; Csizmadia, C.G.; Krom, Y.; Hylkema, H.B.; Van Geel, A.M.; Koopman, H.M.; Verloove-Vanhorick, S.P.; Mearin, M.L. Long-term health and quality-of-life consequences of mass screening for childhood celiac disease: A 10-year follow-up study. *Pediatrics* **2009**, *123*, e582–e588. [CrossRef]
30. Kinos, S.; Kurppa, K.; Ukkola, A.; Collin, P.; Lähdeaho, M.L.; Huhtala, H.; Kekkonen, L.; Mäki, M.; Kaukinen, K. Burden of illness in screen-detected children with celiac disease and their families. *J. Pediatr. Gastroenterol. Nutr.* **2012**, *55*, 412–416. [CrossRef]
31. Oliveira, G.N.; Mohan, R.; Fagbemi, A. Review of celiac disease presentation in a pediatric tertiary centre. *Arq. De Gastroenterol.* **2018**, *55*, 86–93. [CrossRef]
32. Al Sarkhy, A.; El Mouzan, M.I.; Saeed, E.; Alanazi, A.; Alghamdi, S.; Anil, S.; Assiri, A. Clinical characteristics of celiac disease and dietary adherence to gluten-free diet among Saudi children. *J. Pediatr. Gastroenterol. Hepatol. Nutr.* **2015**, *18*, 23–29. [CrossRef]
33. Spijkerman, M.; Tan, I.L.; Kolkman, J.J.; Withoff, S.; Wijmenga, C.; Visschedijk, M.C.; Weersma, R.K. A large variety of clinical features and concomitant disorders in celiac disease—A cohort study in the Netherlands. *Dig. Liver Dis.* **2016**, *48*, 499–505. [CrossRef]
34. Kho, A. Coeliac disease in children in Christchurch, New Zealand: Presentation and patterns from 2000–2010. *World J. Clin. Pediatr.* **2015**, *4*, 148. [CrossRef] [PubMed]
35. Riznik, P.; De Leo, L.; Dolinsek, J.; Gyimesi, J.; Klemenak, M.; Koletzko, B.; Koletzko, S.; Korponay-Szabó, I.R.; Krencnik, T.; Not, T. Clinical Presentation in Children With Coeliac Disease in Central Europe. *J. Pediatr. Gastroenterol. Nutr.* **2021**, *72*, 546–551. [CrossRef] [PubMed]
36. Ravikumara, M.; Nootigattu, V.; Sandhu, B. Ninety Percent of Celiac Disease Is Being Missed. *J. Pediatr. Gastroenterol. Nutr.* **2007**, *45*, 497–499. [CrossRef]
37. Whitburn, J.; Rao, S.R.; Paul, S.P.; Sandhu, B.K. Diagnosis of celiac disease is being missed in over 80% of children particularly in those from socioeconomically deprived backgrounds. *Eur. J. Pediatr.* **2021**, *180*, 1941–1946. [CrossRef]
38. Kvamme, J.M.; Sørbye, S.; Florholmen, J.; Halstensen, T.S. Population-based screening for celiac disease reveals that the majority of patients are undiagnosed and improve on a gluten-free diet. *Sci. Rep.* **2022**, *12*, 12647. [CrossRef]
39. Mårild, K.; Söderling, J.; Bozorg, S.R.; Everhov, Å.H.; Lebwohl, B.; Green, P.H.; Neovius, M.; Ludvigsson, J.F. Costs and Use of Health Care in Patients with Celiac Disease: A Population-Based Longitudinal Study. *Am. J. Gastroenterol.* **2020**, *115*, 1253–1263. [CrossRef] [PubMed]

40. Ukkola, A.; Kurppa, K.; Collin, P.; Huhtala, H.; Forma, L.; Kekkonen, L.; Mäki, M.; Kaukinen, K. Use of health care services and pharmaceutical agents in coeliac disease: A prospective nationwide study. *BMC Gastroenterol.* **2012**, *12*, 136. [CrossRef] [PubMed]
41. Fuchs, V.; Kurppa, K.; Huhtala, H.; Mäki, M.; Kekkonen, L.; Kaukinen, K. Delayed celiac disease diagnosis predisposes to reduced quality of life and incremental use of health care services and medicines: A prospective nationwide study. *United Eur. Gastroenterol. J.* **2018**, *6*, 567–575. [CrossRef]
42. Mattila, E.; Kurppa, K.; Ukkola, A.; Collin, P.; Huhtala, H.; Forma, L.; Lähdeaho, M.L.; Kekkonen, L.; Mäki, M.; Kaukinen, K. Burden of illness and use of health care services before and after celiac disease diagnosis in children. *J. Pediatr. Gastroenterol. Nutr.* **2013**, *57*, 53–56. [CrossRef] [PubMed]
43. Mearns, E.S.; Taylor, A.; Boulanger, T.; Craig, K.J.; Gerber, M.; Leffler, D.A.; Lebwohl, B. Systematic Literature Review of the Economic Burden of Celiac Disease. *Pharmacoeconomics* **2019**, *37*, 45–61. [CrossRef]
44. Norström, F.; Lindholm, L.; Sandström, O.; Nordyke, K.; Ivarsson, A. Delay to celiac disease diagnosis and its implications for health-related quality of life. *BMC Gastroenterol.* **2011**, *11*, 118. [CrossRef] [PubMed]
45. Ludvigsson, J.F.; Card, T.R.; Kaukinen, K.; Bai, J.; Zingone, F.; Sanders, D.S.; Murray, J.A. Screening for celiac disease in the general population and in high-risk groups. *United Eur. Gastroenterol. J.* **2015**, *3*, 106–120. [CrossRef]
46. Norström, F.; Myléus, A.; Nordyke, K.; Carlsson, A.; Högberg, L.; Sandström, O.; Lindholm, L. Is mass screening for coeliac disease a wise use of resources? A health economic evaluation. *BMC Gastroenterol.* **2021**, *21*, 159. [CrossRef]
47. Elwenspoek, M.M.; Thom, H.; Sheppard, A.L.; Keeney, E.; O'Donnell, R.; Jackson, J.; Whiting, P.F. Defining the optimum strategy for identifying adults and children with coeliac disease: Systematic review and economic modelling. *Health Technol. Assess.* **2022**, *26*, 1–310. [CrossRef]
48. Auricchio, R.; Tosco, A.; Piccolo, E.; Galatola, M.; Izzo, V.; Maglio, M.; Greco, L. Potential Celiac Children: 9-Year Follow-Up on a Gluten-Containing Diet. *Am. J. Gastroenterol.* **2014**, *109*, 913–921. [CrossRef]
49. Auricchio, R.; Mandile, R.; Del Vecchio, M.R.; Scapaticci, S.; Galatola, M.; Maglio, M.; Greco, L. Progression of Celiac Disease in Children with Antibodies against Tissue Transglutaminase and Normal Duodenal Architecture. *Gastroenterology* **2019**, *157*, 413–420. [CrossRef]
50. Sakhuja, S.; Holtz, L.R. Progression of pediatric celiac disease from potential celiac disease to celiac disease: A retrospective cohort study. *BMC Pediatr.* **2021**, *21*, 1–7. [CrossRef] [PubMed]
51. Lionetti, E.; Castellaneta, S.; Francavilla, R.; Pulvirenti, A.; Catassi, G.N.; Catassi, C. Long-Term Outcome of Potential Celiac Disease in Genetically at-Risk Children: The Prospective CELIPREV Cohort Study. *J. Clin. Med.* **2019**, *8*, 186. [CrossRef]
52. Sandström, O.; Norström, F.; Carlsson, A.; Högberg, L.; Van der Palz, M.; Stenhammar, L.; Myléus, A. Five-year follow-up of new cases after a coeliac disease mass screening. *Arch. Dis. Child.* **2022**, *107*, 596–600. [CrossRef]
53. Iorfida, D.; Valitutti, F.; Vestri, A.; Di Rocco, A.; Cucchiara, S.; Lubrano, R.; Montuori, M. Dietary Compliance and Quality of Life in Celiac Disease: A Long-Term Follow-Up of Primary School Screening-Detected Patients. *Front. Pediatr.* **2021**, *9*, 787938. [CrossRef]
54. Fabiani, E.; Taccari, L.M.; Rätsch, I.M.; Di Giuseppe, S.; Coppa, G.V.; Catassi, C. Compliance with gluten-free diet in adolescents with screening-detected celiac disease: A 5-year follow-up study. *J. Pediatr.* **2000**, *136*, 841–843. [CrossRef] [PubMed]
55. Germone, M.; Phu, T.; Slosky, C.; Pan, Z.; Jones, A.; Stahl, M.; Mehta, P.; Shull, M.; Ariefdjohan, M.; Liu, E. Anxiety and Depression in Pediatric Patients with Celiac Disease: A Large Cross-Sectional Study. *J. Pediatr. Gastroenterol. Nutr.* **2022**, *75*, 181–185. [CrossRef] [PubMed]
56. Roberts, S.E.; Morrison-Rees, S.; Thapar, N.; Benninga, M.A.; Borrelli, O.; Broekaert, I.; Williams, J.G. Systematic review and meta-analysis: The incidence and prevalence of paediatric coeliac disease across Europe. *Aliment. Pharmacol. Ther.* **2021**, *54*, 109–128. [CrossRef] [PubMed]

nutrients

MDPI

Article

Evaluation of the Usefulness of an Automatable Immunoassay for Monitoring Celiac Disease by Quantification of Immunogenic Gluten Peptides in Urine

Verónica Segura [1,†], Ángela Ruiz-Carnicer [1,†], Irati Mendía [2], Marta Garzón-Benavides [3], Ángeles E. Pizarro [3], Isabel Comino [1] and Carolina Sousa [1,*]

1 Department of Microbiology and Parasitology, Faculty of Pharmacy, University of Seville, 41012 Seville, Spain
2 Biomedal S.L., 41900 Camas, Spain
3 Digestive Disease Clinical Unit, CIBERehd, Institute of Biomedicine of Seville (IBiS), SeLiver Group, Virgen del Rocío Hospital/CSIC/US, 41013 Seville, Spain
* Correspondence: csoumar@us.es
† These authors contributed equally to this work.

Abstract: A gluten-free diet (GFD) is currently the only treatment available for patients with celiac disease (CD). However, adherence to a GFD can be challenging because gluten is present in many foods. A lifelong follow-up of patients with CD must be performed to promote adherence to a GFD and to identify the appearance of symptoms and the associated diseases. Therefore, the development of tools to analyze gluten exposure in these patients is important. This study proposes the development of the first automatable ELISA to monitor adherence to a GFD through the quantification of urine gluten immunogenic peptides (u-GIP). Seven healthy volunteers without suspicion of CD and 23 patients with CD were monitored as part of this study to optimize, validate, and apply this assay. Non-interference was found in the urine matrix, and the recovery percentage for spiked samples was 81–101%. The u-GIP was stable for up to 16 days when the samples were stored at different temperatures. Overall, 100% of the patients had detectable u-GIP at diagnosis (range of 0.39–2.14 ng GIP/mL), which reduced to 27% after 12 months on a GFD. Therefore, this highly sensitive immunoassay would allow the analysis of u-GIP from a large battery of samples in clinical laboratories of specialized healthcare centers.

Keywords: celiac disease; ELISA; gluten-free diet; gluten immunogenic peptides; urine

1. Introduction

Celiac disease (CD) is a systemic disease triggered by the immune system following the ingestion of gluten in genetically predisposed individuals [1,2]. Its prevalence in the general population is approximately 1%, with female predominance. The disease can occur at any age, with a variety of symptoms/manifestations. Exposure to gluten may trigger intestinal symptoms (diarrhea, constipation, abdominal pain, bloating) and/or extraintestinal symptoms (headaches, peripheral neuropathy, dermatitis herpetiformis, gluten ataxia, low bone mineral density, and osteoporosis) [3]. In addition, CD is characterized by an elevation of specific antibodies, such as anti-gliadin and antitissue transglutaminase (anti-tTG), and the presence of HLA-DQ2/DQ8 haplotypes. The only available treatment for CD is a strict lifelong adherence to a gluten-free diet (GFD), which requires significant patient education, motivation, and follow-up. Once a GFD is initiated, the duodenal mucosa begins to heal, and most people report that their symptoms resolve [4]. Despite this improvement in symptoms, a strict GFD must be maintained to prevent ongoing damage to the intestinal tract and symptoms induced by inadvertent gluten ingestion. However, the ubiquitous nature of gluten in food, educational misinformation, inadequate food-labeling regulations, social constraints, and possible cross-contamination of food products make strict adherence to a GFD challenging. Therefore, the GFD represents a challenge, leading scientists to seek alternative or complementary treatments based on non-dietary therapies for CD. Most of the developing therapies are only in the pre-clinical phase, with only a few being tested in phase 2b or 3 trials. Although new approaches raise the hope for coeliacs, giving them a chance to return to gluten, for the time being, a cautionary appraisal of new therapies suggests that they may have a complementary role to gluten withdrawal, mainly to prevent inadvertent gluten contamination [5,6]. Consequently, several studies based on nutritional questionnaires, serological tests, and evaluating gluten immunogenic peptides (GIP) in stool and urine, have reported the non-adherence to a GFD in patients with CD to be between 10 and 88% in adults and between 2–77% in children [7–14]. Furthermore, recent studies have suggested that the persistence of atrophy is due to the recurrence of gluten exposure [15]. Some laboratory tests are available for the evaluation of dietary adherence, and among them, the measurement of GIP levels in urine and stool samples have been highlighted as the most relevant and clinically novel [1,2,16,17]. It is an accurate, reliable, and specific test and a non-invasive technique for the direct detection of gluten ingestion, in contrast to the classical methods, which only detect the consequences of not adhering to a GFD [18–26]. Additionally, concordance has been demonstrated between the absence of GIP excretion and the absence of a histological duodenal lesion [8].

Urine is an advantageous sample for disease monitoring because it can be collected non-invasively, in large amounts, and repeatedly over long periods [27]. However, urine samples are highly heterogeneous matrices with low protein content, making the development of immunoassays for biomarkers detection complicated. Urine contains organic molecules, such as urea, creatinine, and uric acid; inorganic ions such as K^+, Na^+, Cl^-, and Ca^{2+}; cells; as well as peptides of more than 1500 proteins. The concentration of these compounds and the pH usually exhibit considerable variability, not only among individuals, but also between different urine samples taken from the same individual. The complex composition of these samples and its variability, in addition to the high frequency of matrix interferences, complicate the reproducibility and robustness of urine immunoassays [9]. In previous studies, a test for the qualitative measurement of GIP in urine based on a lateral flow immunoassay (LFIA) has been successfully developed [8,9,20]. However, higher throughput solutions are required to obtain quantitative results and analyze a large number of samples. Enzyme-linked immunosorbent assay (ELISA)-based methods can be used to solve these problems. Therefore, the present study aimed to develop the first highly sensitive and automatable method for the quantitative detection of GIP in urine. Here, we describe the optimization, validation, and application of ELISA to quantify GIP in urine samples by monitoring a significant number of patients with CD.

2. Materials and Methods

2.1. Reagents

All of the chemicals were of analytical grade and were used according to the manufacturer's instructions. All of the aqueous solvents and solutions were prepared using double-distilled water. A pure preparation of the horseradish peroxidase conjugates of the G12 (G12-HRP) monoclonal antibody (moAb) and 33-mer peptide (LQLQPF-PQPQLPYPQPQLPYPQPQLPYPQPQPF) was used as the reference standard (Biomedal S.L., Seville, Spain).

2.2. Study Population

A pilot study was conducted, including urine samples from: (1) seven healthy adult volunteers without suspicion of CD and with habitual gluten consumption; (2) seven patients with CD on a strict GFD (previously analyzed by LFIA) to optimize the technique.

In addition, a prospective study including 18 adult patients de novo CD-diagnosed who were recruited between November 2016 and October 2018 was conducted at Virgen del Rocío (Seville, Spain). There were four study visits at diagnosis and 3, 6, and 12 months after diagnosis. The first visit (diagnosis) was at the time of the diagnostic endoscopy, when the patients were untreated (diet with gluten), and at the following visits, they were following a GFD. All participants were instructed by clinical dietitians with experience in CD to follow a GFD. Urine samples were collected at each study visit. The exclusion criteria were: (1) patients who were <14 y old and >80 y old; (2) those with histories of kidney, liver, or severe psychiatric diseases; (3) those with seizure disorders and/or who were currently using anticonvulsants; (4) those who were being treated with long-lasting drugs capable of causing damage to the duodenal mucosa within one year before enrolment. The study protocol was reviewed by the ethics committee of each institution, and written informed consent was obtained from all of the participants.

2.3. *Urine Samples*

2.3.1. Urine Collection

The participants were instructed to collect a 50–100 mL sample of urine in a sealed container and were provided with specific instructions to prevent contamination with gluten during sample collection. The samples were stored at −20 °C until the time of processing.

2.3.2. Spiked Urine Samples

Urine samples from patients with CD on a GFD and GIP negative according to LFIA were spiked with the 33-mer to check for a possible matrix effect and to evaluate recovery. The urine samples were spiked with 0, 1.25, 2.5, 5, 10, and 20 ng/mL of 33-mer peptide and incubated at 4 °C until analysis. The percentage of GIP recovery (R) in the urine was calculated from the average measured (M) and spiked (S) level using the equation $R = (M/S) \times 100$.

2.3.3. Urinary GIP Preconcentration

The urine samples were initially subjected to heat treatment with surfactants. Subsequently, the urine (5 mL) was applied to 3 kDa cutoff centrifugal filtration units (Amicon Ultra-4, UFC800308) and centrifuged. The filtrate was then diluted in the dilution solution used for the ELISA.

2.3.4. Urinary GIP Stability

Three urine samples were collected from three volunteers. Four aliquots of each urine sample were stored at room temperature, 4 °C (refrigerator), and −20 °C (freezer). GIP in the urine was evaluated on days 0, 4, and 16 after collection. The urine samples were tested twice under each condition. To verify the stability of the GIP, the concentration obtained in each urine sample at each time point was compared with the concentration at time 0.

2.4. *Assay Procedure: ELISA*

The ELISA was performed as follows: 96-well microtiter plates (Nunc-Immunoplate Maxisorp, Nunc, Roskilde, Denmark) were coated with G12 moAb. Then, 100 μL of the standard, controls, and urine samples were added in duplicate to the appropriate wells, which were diluted in dilution solution, and the plates were incubated for 60 min at room temperature. Subsequently, the wells were washed five times and incubated with G12-HRP (Biomedal SL, Seville, Spain) dilutions for 1 h at room temperature. Finally, after another washing, 100 μL of enzyme substrate solution (TMB, Sigma Aldrich, St Louis, MO, USA) was added to each well, and the plates were incubated for 30 min in the dark at room temperature. The reaction was stopped with 1M sulfuric acid, and the absorbance was measured at 450 nm (Multiskan SkyHigh; ThermoFisher Scientific, Singapore, Asia).

2.5. *LFIA*

The urine samples were processed according to the manufacturer's recommendations (iVYCHECK GIP Urine; Biomedal S.L., Seville, Spain), and after the processing of the sample, 100 μL of the sample was added onto the detection test strip. This immunochromatographic test uses G12/A1 moAbs and provides a positive if a red/pink line appeared in the result zone of the membrane, providing a signal. The absence suggested a negative result. The blue control line was always used as a test control [5,12,17].

2.6. Statistical Analysis

Statistical analyses were performed using Microsoft® Office Excel (2016), SPSS 25.0 for Windows (SPSS Inc., Chicago, IL, USA) and the Sigma Plot software package (version 12.0; Systat Software, Inc., San Jose, CA, USA). Relative affinity curves were obtained by plotting the maximum absorbance percentage against the reference standard concentration (ng/mL), and EC_{50} was calculated. EC_{50} was defined as the concentration of the line that reduced the maximum absorbance by 50% in the assay. The cross-reactivity (CR) was determined by calculating: (EC_{50} of the standard with the highest antibody affinity/EC_{50} of each tested standard) × 100.

The linearity of the method was established using mobile slope calculations between different points of the line and coefficient correlations (r2). The working range was established between the highest and lowest concentration values with satisfactory accuracy and precision. The acceptance criteria were a coefficient of variation of less than 20% [CV (%) = standard deviation (SD)/mean × 100%]. The slope ($\Delta y/\Delta x$) between points was calculated using the following equation: $\Delta y/\Delta x = (Y1 - Y0)/(X1 - X0)$, Y = concentration (ng/mL 33-mer peptide), and X = absorbance. The limit of quantification (LOQ) was defined as the smallest standard concentration with an intra- and inter-day imprecision lower than 20%. The limit of detection (LOD) of the assay was calculated as follows: mean samples replicates + 3 × SD. A paired Student's t-test was used to analyze the quantitative variables. A p-value < 0.05 was considered statistically significant [28].

3. Results

3.1. Optimization and Validation of the ELISA Working Conditions

The assay was based on a previously developed sandwich ELISA for the analysis of GIP in stools using G12 moAb [21,29]. To obtain a higher sensitivity, new working conditions and applications were determined.

The 33-mer peptide was used as a reference standard, which is one of main contributors to the immunogenicity of gluten [30] and is recognized by the gluten-specific celiac T cells. The influence of different parameters, such as the dilution solution assay, the coating moAb, the curve standard, and the capture moAb concentration, were studied to improve the ELISA conditions for GIP detection in the urine matrix. The optimal concentration of the capture moAb (G12-HRP) was determined using dilutions of 1:100,000 and 1:200,000, with increments of 20,000. For this, six curves with known concentrations of the 33-mer peptide (1–1000 ng/mL 33-mer) were generated (Figure 1A). The 1:100,000 dilution had the lowest EC_{50} of those studied, suggesting that it was more specific for the 33-mer peptide (Figure 1B). Therefore, it was used as the optimal moAb titration in the ELISA.

3.1.1. Linearity and Working Range

To define the working range, the 33-mer peptide standard was serially diluted with the dilution solution to known concentrations (12.5, 6.25, 3.12, 1.56 ng/mL) (Figure 2B). Each concentration was tested five times in duplicate. Furthermore, it was performed on different plates, on different days, and by different analysts to demonstrate, in turn, the robustness of the assay.

The coefficient of variation (CV%) for the same concentrations was below 20% in the tested standards, ensuring the good precision and robustness of the method. Similarly, the CV between consecutive standards had a CV% between 20–80%, showing the correct discrimination among the consecutive standards, until the 12.5 ng/mL concentration.

In this type of assay, the approximation of the different standard values is carried out in a polynomial manner (curve), and the slope ($\Delta y/\Delta x$) between the two concentrations of two contiguous points was determined (12.5–6.25, 6.25–3.12, and 3.12–1.56 ng/mL). The slope ($\Delta y/\Delta x$) between points was calculated using the following equation: $\Delta y/\Delta x = (Y1 - Y0)/(X1 - X0)$, Y = concentration (ng/mL 33-mer peptide), and X = absorbance (Figure 2A). Subsequently, the CV% of the different slopes ($\Delta y/\Delta x$) between the different concentrations was calculated and found to be constant, not exceeding 20% [28].

A

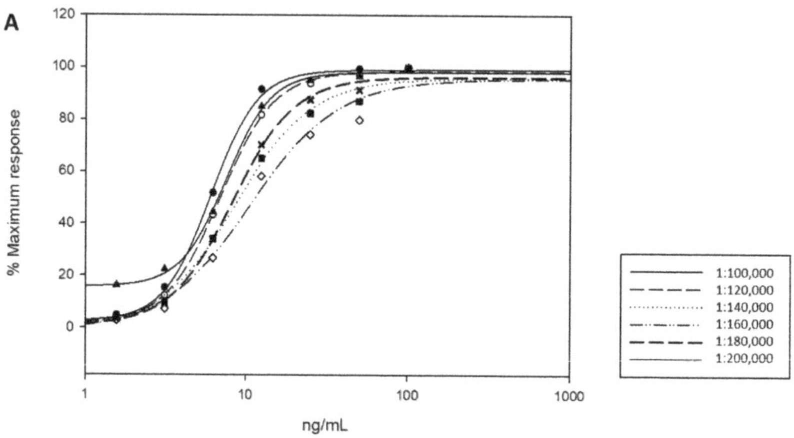

B

[G12-HRP]	EC_{50} (ng/mL)	%CR
1:100,000	6.1	100
1:120,000	7.0	87.1
1:140,000	8.7	69.2
1:160,000	10.7	56.5
1:180,000	8.3	72.9
1:200,000	7.5	80.4

Figure 1. G12-HRP moAb titration for sandwich ELISA optimization. (**A**). Relative affinity of G12-HRP moAb for 33-mer peptide. (**B**). Standard reference curves. EC_{50} and cross-reactivity (CR) were obtained by G12 ELISA. EC_{50} is the line concentration that reduces the maximum absorbance by 50% in the assay. CR was calculated as follows: (EC_{50} of the antigen for which the moAb was raised/EC_{50} of each antigen assayed) $\times$ 100. These assays were performed in duplicate moAb, monoclonal antibody.

In addition, the regression coefficient was calculated from the polynomial approximation of the analyzed standards, and it was verified that there were no statistically significant differences between the curves (correlation coefficient (r2) > 0.99) (Figure 2C).

3.1.2. Matrix Study

A common challenge in immunoassays is matrix interference. These interferences can be reduced by dilution or by using a matrix-matched calibration curve. Therefore, the behavior of the 33-mer peptide standard was evaluated in the dilution solution and the urine matrix. Urine samples from a patient with CD on a GFD strictly controlled by a dietary questionnaire and previously analyzed by LFIA with negative results, were used. Twelve curves with known concentrations of the 33-mer peptide (12.5, 6.25, 3.12, and 1.56 ng/mL) were performed. The CV% for the same concentration in each matrix showed <20%. A comparison of the spiked curves (in dilution solution or urine) did not show a statistically significant difference ($p > 0.1$). Thus, the ELISA detected only the 33-mer peptide without any interference from the dilution solution or urine matrix (Figure 3).

A

Standard curve	Concentration (ng/mL) 12.5 (Y_1) Abs (X_1)	Concentration (ng/mL) 6.25 (Y_0) Abs (X_0)	Δy/Δx (12.5-6.25 ng/mL)	Concentration (ng/mL) 6.25 (Y_1) Abs (X_1)	Concentration (ng/mL) 3.12 (Y_0) Abs (X_0)	Δy/Δx (6.25-3.12 ng/mL)	Concentration (ng/mL) 3.12 (Y_1) Abs (X_1)	Concentration (ng/mL) 1.56 (Y_0) Abs (X_0)	Δy/Δx (3.12-1.56 ng/mL)
Standard curve 1	2.799	1.633	5.360	1.633	0.503	2.769	0.503	0.118	4.057
Standard curve 2	3.166	1.303	3.355	1.303	0.421	3.549	0.421	0.098	4.830
Standard curve 3	2.513	1.185	4.705	1.185	0.308	3.571	0.308	0.066	6.433
Standard curve 4	3.257	1.619	3.816	1.619	0.394	2.554	0.394	0.099	5.288
Standard curve 5	3.169	1.727	4.336	1.727	0.478	2.505	0.478	0.120	4.364
		Mean	4.314		Mean	2.990		Mean	4.994
		SD	0.777		SD	0.530		SD	0.930
		CV%	18		CV%	18		CV%	19

B

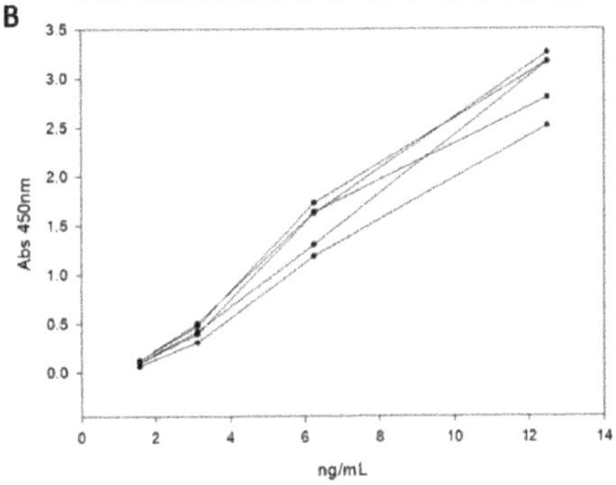

C

Standard curve	Correlation coefficient (r^2)
Standard curve 1	0.997
Standard curve 2	0.995
Standard curve 3	0.995
Standard curve 4	0.999
Standard curve 5	0.995

Figure 2. (**A**) Calculation of slopes (Δy/Δx) between the different concentrations of the curve and the correlation coefficient (r2). The slope (Δy/Δx) between concentrations was calculated using the equation; Δy/Δx = (Y1 − Y0)/(X1 − X0); Y = concentration (ng/mL 33-mer), and X = absorbance. (**B**). Polynomial representation of 33-mer concentrations (12.5 and 1.56 ng/mL). (**C**). Correlation coefficient (r2) calculated from the polynomial approximation of the standards analyzed. Abs, absorbance; CV%, coefficient of variation; SD, standard deviation.

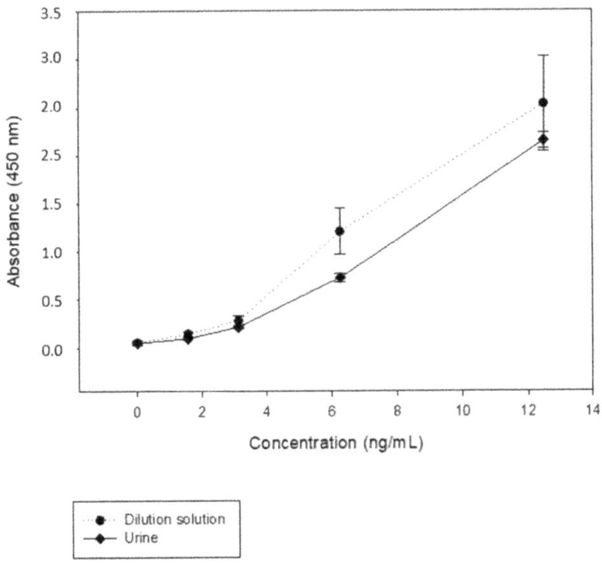

Figure 3. Standard curve for the quantification of the 33-mer used as reference material. The linear portion of the curve is between 12.5 and 1.56 ng/mL. The solid black line represents the mean values and standard deviations (SD) of 12 determinations per concentration in the urine matrix and the dashed line in the dilution solution.

3.1.3. Accuracy and Precision

The most useful method for calculating the accuracy was the recovery test using three different concentrations. The Association of Official Agricultural Chemists (AOAC) has established an optimal recovery percentage for spiked samples of 80% to 120% [31]. According to this criterion, the recovery (%R) of all the spiked samples was satisfactory using this method. All of the non-spiked samples were below the LOQ. According to the Eurachem guide [28], the results must be obtained from an average of 6–15 replicates of each material, with the same equipment, analyst, and laboratory, and in a short period [28]. In this study, the accuracy was calculated by taking nine measurements per concentration (20, 10, 5, 2.5, 1,25 ng/mL of 33-mer peptide), and these measurements were made on the same day. The results indicated an accuracy of 91% on day one and 89% on day two. In addition, to calculate the precision, nine replicates were made by concentrations on two different days, obtaining a precision of 90% (Table 1).

Table 1. Analysis of the spiked urine samples by sandwich ELISA. Results are expressed as ng/mL of 33-mer (mean ± SD) and percentage of recovery (R). N = number of analyses; <LOQ, less than the limit of quantification; SD, standard deviation.

	Spiked Sample (ng/mL)	N	ng/mL ± SD	% R	Accuracy (%)	Precision (%)
Day 1	20.0	9	20.3 ± 3.3	101	91%	90%
	10.0	9	8.1 ± 0.5	81		
	5.0	9	4.6 ± 0.4	91		
	2.5	9	<LOQ			
	1.25	9	<LOQ			
	0	9	<LOQ			
Day 2	20.0	9	17.8 ± 2.8	89	89%	
	10.0	9	8.2 ± 0.6	82		
	5.0	9	4.8 ± 0.3	96		
	2.5	9	<LOQ			
	1.25	9	<LOQ			
	0	9	<LOQ			

3.2. *Effect of the Urine Samples on the Assay Performance*

To evaluate the usefulness of the developed method, seven adult volunteers without suspicion of CD and seven patients with CD on a GFD strictly controlled by a dietary questionnaire were recruited into a pilot study. These samples were previously analyzed by LFIA and showed positive results in the volunteers without suspected CD and negative results in the patients with CD. The urine samples were subjected to extraction and concentration. The urine samples were mixed with surfactant agents and incubated in a thermostatic bath. The sample was passed through a 3 kDa filter and centrifuged. Once the samples were obtained, they were diluted in the dilution solution, and a G12-G12 sandwich ELISA was performed.

The results showed that 100% (7/7) of the subjects without CD were GIP positive, with values between 0.40 and 1.01 ng GIP/mL of urine. However, the urine samples from the patients with CD on a GFD were negative for GIP (<LOQ). Considering these results, the LOQ was established as 0.312 ng GIP/mL of urine with a concentration factor of 10, and a dilution factor of 2. The LOQ was determined to be reliable because it was also found to be above the LOD of this procedure. The LOD, calculated as the mean of seven GIP negative sample replicates + 3 SD, was 0.075 ng GIP/mL of urine.

3.3. *Stability of GIP*

Conditions that allow the storage/accumulation of urine samples over time, without loss of the GIP signal, were studied to allow for the bulk analysis of urine samples. The storage and transport temperature conditions of the samples should be adequate to guarantee the stability of GIP in the urine. A stability study was carried out with three volunteers: two healthy adult volunteers without suspicion of CD (volunteers 1 and 2) and a patient with CD on a strict GFD (volunteer 3). Four aliquots of each urine sample were stored at room temperature, 4 °C and −20 °C. The GIP in the urine was evaluated on days 0, 4 and 16 after collection. The urines were tested twice in each condition. To check the stability of the GIP in the urine, each condition was compared with the time point t0, by executing at least two determinations per condition. Our results showed that urinary GIP is stable for up to 16 days when the samples are stored at different temperature conditions (room temperature, 4 °C, and −20 °C) according to the sandwich ELISA (deviation below 20% of the expected value) (Figure 4).

A

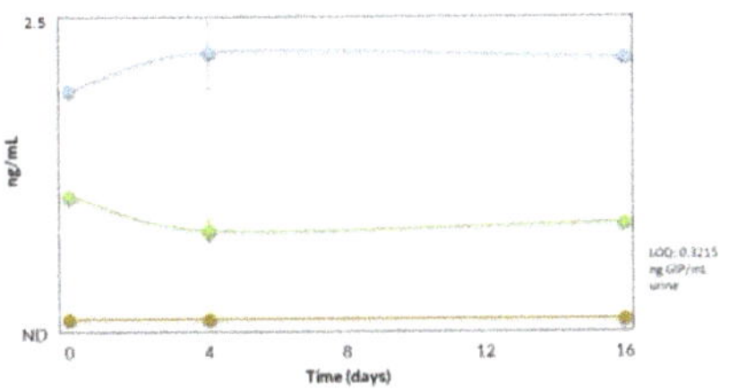

Room temperature					
	Time (days)				
	0	4	16	CV%	
Volunteer	ng GIP/mL	ng GIP/mL	ng GIP/mL	t0-t4	t0-t16
1	1.48±0.37	1.96±0.48	1.88±0.07	20%	17%
2	0.67±0.09	0.52±0.04	0.55±0.01	18%	14%
3	<LOQ	<LOQ	<LOQ	n/a	n/a

B

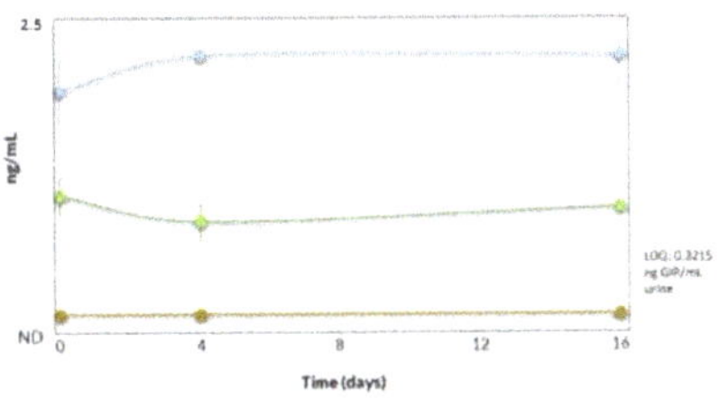

4°C temperature					
	Time (days)				
	0	4	16	CV%	
Volunteer	ng GIP/mL	ng GIP/mL	ng GIP/mL	t0-t4	t0-t16
1	1.48±0.37	1.93±0.20	1.93±0.40	19%	19%
2	0.67±0.09	0.55±0.07	0.61±0.02	14%	7%
3	<LOQ	<LOQ	<LOQ	n/a	n/a

C

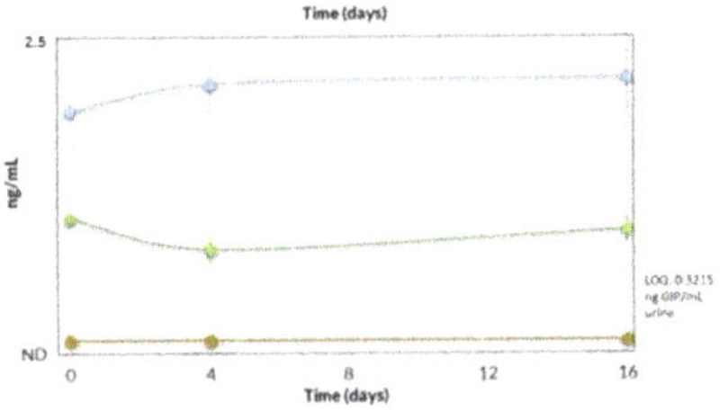

-20°C temperature					
	Time (days)				
	0	4	16	CV%	
Volunteer	ng GIP/mL	ng GIP/mL	ng GIP/mL	t0-t4	t0-t16
1	1.48±0.37	1.8±0.34	1.88±0.40	14%	17%
2	0.67±0.09	0.53±0.05	0.61±0.06	16%	7%
3	<LOQ	<LOQ	<LOQ	n/a	n/a

Figure 4. Stability of urinary GIP over a 16-day period. (**A**) room temperature. (**B**) 4 °C. (**C**) −20 °C. Volunteer one is represented in blue, two in green, and three in yellow. Each point represents the mean of duplicate measurements plus the SD if the GIP was measurable. GIP, gluten immunogenic peptides; LOQ, limit of quantification; ND, non-determined; n/a, non-applied.

4. Clinical Study

4.1. *Study Design and Population*

The study population consisted of 12 (67%) females and six (33%) males, with a median age of 42 years. Table 2 presents the descriptive data of the patients; 72% of the patients started the study because of the presence of symptoms, 94% were seropositive (CD antibodies) at diagnosis, and the most common histological lesion was Marsh II-III (89%). Participant retention was 72% at three months, 72% at six months, and 61% at 12 months (the most common reason for being lost to follow-up was moving out of the study area, not attending follow-up visits, and forgetting to collect samples).

Table 2. Characteristics of the patients enrolled in the study. CD, celiac disease.

Characteristics	Patients, n	%
Sex		
Female	12	67
Male	6	33
Age		
Median age (42)		
Duodenal histology		
Marsh 0-I	2	11
Marsh II-III	16	89
Symptoms		
Asymptomatic	5	28
Symptomatic	13	72
CD antibodies		
CD antibodies positive	17	94
CD antibodies negative	1	6

4.2. Analysis of Urine GIP

At the initial visit, before starting the GFD, 100% (18/18) of the patients had detectable GIP in the provided urine sample, with a range of 0.39 and 2.14 ng GIP/mL of urine. After diagnosis and treatment with a GFD, the rate of GIP positive urine was 38% at three months, 38% at six months, and 27% at 12 months, and in general, the GIP concentration in those urine samples also decreased. In particular, the GFD compliance rates increased as the study progressed (Figure 5A,B). Therefore, significant differences in the GIP excretion levels were observed in the population before and after the GFD initiation, as shown in Figure 5. These results were comparable to those obtained in a pediatric population at the follow-up of two years reported by Comino et al. [29], in which fecal GIP was evaluated by ELISA G12. Therefore, a study is currently underway in a pediatric population to corroborate these results.

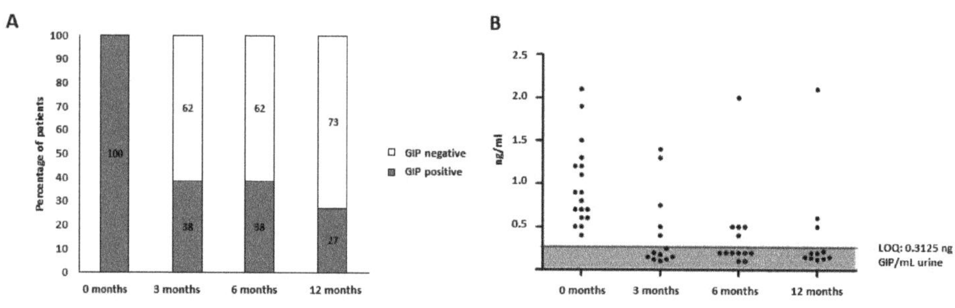

Figure 5. Concentration of urine GIP from patients with CD at the baseline visit and over 12 months after the initiation of a GFD. (**A**) Percentage distribution of the GFD-treated patients with CD according to GIP concentration. (**B**) GIP levels in urine at the basal and follow-up visits (basal, three, six, and 12 months). CD, celiac disease; GFD, gluten-free diet; GIP, gluten immunogenic peptides; LOQ, limit of quantification.

5. Conclusions

We propose the first automated and highly sensitive method for the quantitative detection of GIP in urine for the monitoring of CD. In this study, several parameters were optimized to obtain a reproducible, selective, and sensitive method. Additionally, this method demonstrated the feasibility of clearly identifying gluten consumption by measuring multiple urine samples from healthy adult volunteers with habitual consumption of gluten, and from patients with CD on a strict GFD. Furthermore, a small prospective clinical study was carried out and the results showed statistically significant differences in the determination of GIP in urine between individuals at CD diagnosis and follow-up. As the presence of u-GIP is direct evidence that gluten intake has occurred, this method could either be used to evaluate the adherence to a GFD or for the confirmation of gluten intake in cases where a gluten challenge is necessary, such as for confirmation of the disease or in clinical trials where CD drugs are being tested. However, further studies with larger numbers of pediatric and adult patients are needed to support the study findings for the implementation of this new method in the clinical laboratories of specialized health centers. In addition, interlaboratory trial studies would be required to establish the efficacy and comparability of the new method, as well as to validate the uncertainty estimates indicated.

Author Contributions: Conceptualization, V.S., Á.R.-C., I.M., M.G.-B., Á.E.P., I.C. and C.S.; Data curation, V.S., Á.R.-C., I.M., I.C. and C.S.; Formal analysis, V.S., Á.R.-C., I.M., I.C. and C.S.; Funding acquisition, I.C. and C.S.; Investigation, V.S., Á.R.-C., I.M., M.G.-B., Á.E.P., I.C. and C.S.; Methodology, V.S., Á.R.-C. and I.M.; Project administration, I.C. and C.S.; Resources, I.C. and C.S.; Software, V.S. and Á.R.-C.; Supervision, I.C. and C.S.; Validation, I.C. and C.S.; Visualization, I.C. and C.S.; Writing—original draft, V.S., Á.R.-C., I.C. and C.S.; Writing—review and editing, V.S., Á.R.-C., I.M., M.G.-B., Á.E.P., I.C. and C.S. All authors have read and agreed to the published version of the manuscript.

Funding: This research was funded by Grant DI-17-09627 and Grant RTC2019-006806-1 funded by MCIN/AEI/10.13039/501100011033, by Grant P18-RT-3004 funded by PAIDI I+D+i Junta de Andalucía (Consejería de Economía y Conocimiento), and by Grant AT17_5489_USE PAIDI Actividades de Transferencia 2017 Junta de Andalucía (Consejería de Economía, Conocimiento, Empresas y Universidad).

Institutional Review Board Statement: The study protocol was reviewed by the ethics committee of each institution. CEI de los Hospitales Universitarios Virgen Macarena-Virgen del Rocío (Seville, Spain).

Informed Consent Statement: Informed consent was obtained from all of the subjects involved in the study.

Data Availability Statement: Data sharing is not applicable to this article.

Conflicts of Interest: Author Irati Mendíaz is employed by the company Biomedal S.L. The contribution of the author in the paper is participation in the experimental design. However, the Biomedal S.L. company did not contribute financially. Therefore, there is no conflict of interest in relation to the Biomedal S.L., company. The remaining authors declare that the research was conducted in the absence of any commercial or financial relationships that could be construed as a potential conflict of interest.

References

1. Al-Toma, A.; Volta, U.; Auricchio, R.; Castillejo, G.; Sanders, D.S.; Cellier, C.; Mulder, C.J.; Lundin, K.E.A. European Society for the Study of Coeliac Disease (ESsCD) guideline for coeliac disease and other gluten-related disorders. *United Eur. Gastroenterol. J.* **2019**, *7*, 583–613. [CrossRef]
2. Husby, S.; Koletzko, S.; Korponay-Szabó, I.; Kurppa, K.; Mearin, M.L.; Ribes-Koninckx, C.; Shamir, R.; Troncone, R.; Auricchio, R.; Castillejo, G.; et al. European Society Paediatric Gastroenterology, Hepatology and Nutrition Guidelines for Diagnosing Coeliac Disease 2020. *J. Pediatr. Gastroenterol. Nutr.* **2020**, *70*, 141–156. [CrossRef]
3. Lungaro, L.; Manza, F.; Costanzini, A.; Barbalinardo, M.; Gentili, D.; Caputo, F.; Guarino, M.; Zoli, G.; Volta, U.; De Giorgio, R.; et al. Osteoporosis and celiac disease: Updates and hidden pitfalls. *Nutrients* **2023**, *15*, 1089. [CrossRef] [PubMed]
4. Ludvigsson, J.F.; Bai, J.C.; Biagi, F.; Card, T.R.; Ciacci, C.; Ciclitira, P.J.; Green, P.H.; Hadjivassiliou, M.; Holdoway, A.; van Heel, D.A.; et al. BSG Coeliac Disease Guidelines Development Group; British Society of Gastroenterology. Diagnosis and management of adult coeliac disease: Guidelines from the British Society of Gastroenterology. *Gut* **2014**, *63*, 1210–1228. [CrossRef] [PubMed]
5. Caio, G.; Ciccocioppo, R.; Zoli, G.; De Giorgio, R.; Volta, U. Therapeutic options for coeliac disease: What else beyond gluten-free diet? *Dig. Liver Dis.* **2020**, *52*, 130–137. [CrossRef] [PubMed]
6. Caio, G.; Volta, U.; Sapone, A.; Leffler, D.A.; De Giorgio, R.; Catassi, C.; Fasano, A. Celiac disease: A comprehensive current review. *BMC Med.* **2019**, *17*, 142. [CrossRef]
7. Muhammad, H.; Reeves, S.; Jeanes, Y.M. Identifying and improving adherence to the gluten-free diet in people with coeliac disease. *Proc. Nutr. Soc.* **2019**, *78*, 418–425. [CrossRef] [PubMed]

8. Ruiz-Carnicer, Á.; Garzón-Benavides, M.; Fombuena, B.; Segura, V.; García-Fernández, F.; Sobrino-Rodríguez, S.; Gómez-Izquierdo, L.; Montes-Cano, M.A.; Rodríguez-Herrera, A.; Millán, R.; et al. Negative predictive value of the repeated absence of gluten immunogenic peptides in the urine of treated celiac patients in predicting mucosal healing: New proposals for follow-up in celiac disease. *Am. J. Clin. Nutr.* **2020**, *112*, 1240–1251. [CrossRef]
9. Coto, L.; Mendia, I.; Sousa, C.; Bai, J.C.; Cebolla, A. Determination of gluten immunogenic peptides for the management of the treatment adherence of celiac disease: A systematic review. *World J. Gastroenterol.* **2021**, *27*, 6306–6321. [CrossRef]
10. Stefanolo, J.P.; Tálamo, M.; Dodds, S.; de la Paz Temprano, M.; Costa, A.F.; Moreno, M.L.; Pinto-Sánchez, M.I.; Smecuol, E.; Vázquez, H.; Gonzalez, A.; et al. Real-World gluten exposure in patients with celiac disease on gluten-free diets, determined from gliadin immunogenic peptides in urine and fecal samples. *Clin. Gastroenterol. Hepatol.* **2021**, *19*, 484–491.e1. [CrossRef]
11. Segura, V.; Ruiz-Carnicer, Á.; Sousa, C.; Moreno, M.L. New insights into non-dietary treatment in celiac disease: Emerging therapeutic options. *Nutrients* **2021**, *13*, 2146. [CrossRef] [PubMed]
12. Wieser, H.; Ruiz-Carnicer, Á.; Segura, V.; Comino, I.; Sousa, C. Challenges of monitoring the gluten-free diet adherence in the management and follow-up of patients with celiac disease. *Nutrients* **2021**, *13*, 2274. [CrossRef]
13. Sandström, O.; Norström, F.; Carlsson, A.; Högberg, L.; van der Palz, M.; Stenhammar, L.; Webb, C.; Ivarsson, A.; Myléus, A. Five-year follow-up of new cases after a coeliac disease mass screening. *Arch. Dis. Child.* **2022**, *107*, 596–600. [CrossRef] [PubMed]
14. Machado, M.V. New Developments in celiac disease treatment. *Int. J. Mol. Sci.* **2023**, *24*, 945. [CrossRef]
15. Garzón-Benavides, M.; Ruiz-Carnicer, Á.; Segura, V.; Fombuena, B.; García-Fernandez, F.; Sobrino-Rodriguez, S.; Gómez-Izquierdo, L.; Montes-Cano, M.A.; Millan-Domínguez, R.; María del Carmen Rico, M.; et al. Regular monitoring of patients with coeliac disease by determinations of gluten immunogenic peptides in urine improved gluten-free diet adherence and the healing of duodenal mucosa: Proposal on a new algorithm for the follow-up of coeliac disease. *Aliment. Pharmacol. Ther.* **2023**, in press.
16. Rodrigo, L.; Beteta-Gorriti, V.; Alvarez, N.; Gómez de Castro, C.; de Dios, A.; Palacios, L.; Santos-Juanes, J. Cutaneous and mucosal manifestations associated with celiac disease. *Nutrients* **2018**, *10*, 800. [CrossRef]
17. Protocolo Para el Diagnóstico Precoz de la Enfermedad Celíaca. Available online: https://www3.gobiernodecanarias.org/sanidad/scs/contenidoGenerico.jsp?idDocument=ed8e95ff-578d-11e8-8844-65f683d38a9e&idCarpeta=0428f5bb-8968-11dd-b7e9-158e12a49309 (accessed on 10 December 2022).
18. Comino, I.; Real, A.; Vivas, S.; Síglez, M.Á.; Caminero, A.; Nistal, E.; Casqueiro, J.; Rodríguez-Herrera, A.; Cebolla, A.; Sousa, C. Monitoring of gluten-free diet compliance in celiac patients by assessment of gliadin 33-mer equivalent epitopes in feces. *Am. J. Clin. Nutr.* **2012**, *95*, 670–677. [CrossRef] [PubMed]
19. Soler, M.; Estevez, M.C.; del Moreno, M.; Cebolla, A.; Lechuga, L.M. Label-free SPR detection of gluten peptides in urine for non-invasive celiac disease follow-up. *Biosens. Bioelectron.* **2016**, *79*, 158–164. [CrossRef]
20. Moreno, M.D.L.; Cebolla, Á.; Munõz-Suano, A.; Carrillo-Carrion, C.; Comino, I.; Pizarro, Á.; León, F.; Rodríguez-Herrera, A.; Sousa, C. Detection of gluten immunogenic peptides in the urine of patients with coeliac disease reveals transgressions in the gluten-free diet and incomplete mucosal healing. *Gut* **2017**, *66*, 250–257. [CrossRef]
21. Comino, I.; Fernández-Bañares, F.; Esteve, M.; Ortigosa, L.; Castillejo, G.; Fambuena, B.; Ribes-Koninckx, C.; Sierra, C.; Rodríguez-Herrera, A.; Salazar, J.C.; et al. Fecal gluten peptides reveal limitations of serological tests and food questionnaires for monitoring gluten-free diet in celiac disease patients. *Am. J. Gastroenterol.* **2016**, *111*, 1456–1465. [CrossRef]
22. Gerasimidis, K.; Zafeiropoulou, K.; Mackinder, M.; Ijaz, U.Z.; Duncan, H.; Buchanan, E.; Cardigan, T.; Edwards, C.A.; McGrogan, P.; Russell, R.K. Comparison of clinical methods with the faecal gluten immunogenic peptide to assess gluten intake in coeliac disease. *J. Pediatr. Gastroenterol. Nutr.* **2018**, *67*, 356–360. [CrossRef] [PubMed]
23. Peláez, E.C.; Estevez, M.C.; Domínguez, R.; Sousa, C.; Cebolla, A.; Lechuga, L.M. A compact SPR biosensor device for the rapid and efficient monitoring of gluten-free diet directly in human urine. *Anal. Bioanal. Chem.* **2020**, *412*, 6407–6417. [CrossRef] [PubMed]
24. Porcelli, B.; Ferretti, F.; Biviano, I.; Santini, A.; Cinci, F.; Vascotto, M.; Grande, E.; Quagliarella, F.; Terzuoli, L.; Bizzaro, N.; et al. Testing for fecal gluten immunogenic peptides: A useful tool to evaluate compliance with gluten-free diet by celiacs. *Ann. Gastroenterol.* **2020**, *33*, 631–637. [CrossRef] [PubMed]
25. Porcelli, B.; Ferretti, F.; Cinci, F.; Biviano, I.; Santini, A.; Grande, E.; Quagliarella, F.; Terzuoli, L.; Bacarelli, M.R.; Bizzaro, N.; et al. Fecal gluten immunogenic peptides as indicators of dietary compliance in celiac patients. *Minerva Gastroenterol. Dietol.* **2020**, *66*, 201–207. [CrossRef]
26. Fernández-Bañares, F.; Beltrán, B.; Salas, A.; Comino, I.; Ballester-Clau, R.; Ferrer, C.; Molina-Infante, J.; Rosinach, M.; Modolell, I.; Rodríguez-Moranta, F.; et al. Persistent villous atrophy in de novo adult patients with celiac disease and strict control of gluten-free diet adherence: A multicenter prospective study (CADER Study). *Am. J. Gastroenterol.* **2021**, *116*, 1036–1043. [CrossRef]
27. Adachi, J.; Kumar, C.; Zhang, Y.; Olsen, J.V.; Mann, M. The human urinary proteome contains more than 1500 proteins, including a large proportion of membrane proteins. *Genome Biol.* **2006**, *7*, R80. [CrossRef]
28. Magnusson, B.; Örnemark, U. (Eds.) *Eurachem Guide: The Fitness for Purpose of Analytical Methods—A Laboratory Guide to Method Validation and Related Topics*, 2nd ed.; Eurachem: Gembloux, Belgium, 2014; ISBN 978-91-87461-59-0. Available online: www.eurachem.org (accessed on 10 December 2022).
29. Comino, I.; Segura, V.; Ortigosa, L.; Espín, B.; Castillejo, G.; Garrote, J.A.; Sierra, C.; Millán, A.; Ribes-Koninckx, C.; Román, E.; et al. Prospective longitudinal study: Use of faecal gluten immunogenic peptides to monitor children diagnosed with coeliac disease during transition to a gluten-free diet. *Aliment. Pharmacol. Ther.* **2019**, *49*, 1484–1492. [CrossRef]

30. Shan, L.; Molberg, Ø.; Parrot, I.; Hausch, F.; Filiz, F.; Gray, G.M.; Sollid, L.M.; Khosla, C. Structural basis for gluten intolerance in celiac sprue. *Science* **2002**, *297*, 2275–2279. [CrossRef]
31. Abbott, M.; Hayward, S.; Ross, W.; Godefroy, S.B.; Ulberth, F.; Van Hengel, A.J.; Roberts, J.; Akiyama, H.; Popping, B.; Yeung, J.M.; et al. Validation procedures for quantitative food allergen ELISA methods: Community Guidance and Best Practices. *J. AOAC Int.* **2010**, *93*, 442–445. [CrossRef]

nutrients

MDPI

Article

The Importance of an Early Evaluation after Establishing a Gluten-Free Diet in Children with Celiac Disease

Rafael Martín-Masot [1,2], María Jiménez-Muñoz [1], Marta Herrador-López [1], Marta Flor-Alemany [2,3,*], Víctor Manuel Navas-López [1] and Teresa Nestares [2,3]

1 Pediatric Gastroenterology and Nutrition Unit, Hospital Regional Universitario de Malaga, 29010 Málaga, Spain
2 Institute of Nutrition and Food Technology "José MataixVerdú" (INYTA), Biomedical Research Centre (CIBM), University of Granada, 18071 Granada, Spain
3 Department of Physiology, Faculty of Pharmacy, University of Granada, 18071 Granada, Spain
* Correspondence: floralemany@ugr.es

Abstract: A gluten-free diet (GFD) is the only treatment available for celiac disease (CD); hence, it is important to ensure correct adherence to the diet and adequate monitoring of the diet. The present study aims to assess the importance of an early follow-up of celiac patients after diagnosis of the disease, identify the role of stool gluten immunogenic peptides (GIPs) in the assessment of GFD adherence, and analyze possible nutritional imbalances or deficiencies in the GFD. This is a cross-sectional study carried out in pediatric patients with newly diagnosed CD in a tertiary hospital in Spain. Of the 61 patients included, 14% had positive stool GIPS at 4 months after CD diagnosis, Among them, 88% had negative stool GIPS at 9 months after diagnosis, following dietary advice. We found nutritional deficiencies in the GFD, such as vitamin D (with only 27% of patients with adequate intakes), folate, calcium, magnesium, and fiber. Similarly, we found imbalances: excess protein and fat intakes and a high percentage of total daily energy intake came from ultra-processed foods (UPF). These findings emphasize the importance of early follow-up of children after diagnosis of CD. It is also crucial to identify patients with poor GFD compliance based on stool GIPS and analyze GFD nutritional imbalances and deficits. Our findings may contribute to the development of specific strategies for the early follow-up of patients with CD, including appropriate nutritional counselling.

Keywords: celiac disease; gluten-free diet; gluten immunogenic peptides; ultra-processed foods

1. Introduction

Celiac disease (CD) is an immune-mediated systemic pathology, which appears and develops from the dysfunctional interaction between genetic and environmental factors [1]. It is characterized by damage of varying intensity in the duodenal mucosa and a heterogeneous combination of gastrointestinal and/or extraintestinal symptoms, with a prevalence of approximately 1.4% of the population [2–4] and an increasing incidence worldwide [5].

A strict lifelong gluten-free diet (GFD) is the only treatment currently available for CD patients. However, adherence to the GFD is difficult due to the large number of gluten-containing products and cross-contamination [6]. Socioeconomic aspects also play an important role. These factors lead to minimal adherence rates of up to 23% of children [7] and 53% of adults with CD [8]. Some studies in adults [9] have shown a high percentage (approximately 20%) of patients with non-responsive CD, and this is largely due to poor adherence to the GFD. Non-compliance with the GFD may contribute, in addition to enteropathy and, in some cases, persistent symptoms, to the development of diseases with high morbidity and high health and social costs, such as autoimmune diseases, osteopenia/osteoporosis, infertility, repeated miscarriages, neurological/psychiatric disorders, and cancer (especially of the gastrointestinal tract) [2,3,10].

Proper GFD monitoring is crucial, especially in the first year after diagnosis of the CD when adherence to GFD is essential for mucosal recovery. However, there are no firm recommendations on the most efficient method to assess adherence to GFD [11]. Once the GFD is established, traditional methods' sensitivity (clinical, dietary records, and serological tests) decreases markedly to detect persistent mucosal damage [12] and may be ineffective in revealing dietary transgressions or the ingestion of trace of gluten [3]. Duodenal biopsies are reserved for refractory cases due to their invasiveness and cost.

This fact has led to the exploration of more sensitive methods for detecting dietary transgressions, and the multiple determination of gluten immunogenic peptides (GIPs) in biological samples (urine and/or stool) has emerged in this context [13]. GIPs are resistant to gastrointestinal digestion, and part of them can be absorbed into the bloodstream and subsequently excreted in the urine, so that their presence can be determined in urine and stool [14,15] within 6–12 h and 3–5 days, respectively, after gluten ingestion in a normal diet [16]. This non-invasive method provides direct information on recent gluten exposure [10]. Previous studies have evaluated its importance not only as a suitable method for detecting refractory CD [17] but also as a tool for monitoring adherence to GFD [18]. The presence of repeated positive GIPS over several days has been correlated with intestinal mucosal damage [19]. Moreover, its assessment in conjunction with a dietary record concomitant with sample collection allows targeted dietary interventions to be developed during patient follow-up [15,20,21].

The nutritional adequacy of GFD is a controversial issue, as the exclusion of gluten-containing cereals from the diet may lead to deficiencies in the B vitamin group, folic acid, fiber, and vitamin D [22]. Other notable deficiencies include magnesium, calcium, iron, and zinc deficiencies [22]. Therefore, nutritional deficiencies may be due not only to malabsorption caused by the disease itself but also to the characteristics of an inadequate GFD [23]. Recent studies [24] have shown that celiac patients have higher intakes of total fat and added sugars; however, it is unclear whether they have higher intakes of total energy. Most of the studies carried out so far [22,24,25] analyze GFD nutritional imbalances and deficits in the medium and long-term follow-up of patients with CD, and there is still a certain lack of knowledge about the nutritional adequacy and the best follow-up strategy of the GFD in newly diagnosed patients with CD. The nutritional imbalances that have been described in several studies [22–24] indicate that an early approach to the GFD follow-up could be essential, and it is necessary to establish the ideal time to initiate follow-up after diagnosis of the CD.

Consequently, the aims of the present study were to evaluate the importance of an early CD follow-up: (1) determine the adherence to the GFD in recently diagnosed patients with CD and (2) analyze possible nutritional imbalances or deficiencies of the GFD.

2. Materials and Methods

2.1. Subjects

A total of 61 children aged between 2 and 14 years with CD were included in the present cross-sectional pilot study. Participants were recruited from January 2021 to July 2022; children were diagnosed with CD according to the criteria of the European Society of Pediatric Gastroenterology Hepatology and Nutrition (ESPGHAN) [11] and received care at the Pediatric Gastroenterology and Nutrition Unit of the Hospital Regional Universitario in Malaga, Spain. Exclusion criteria were liver or kidney disease, acute and chronic inflammation, inflammatory bowel disease, diabetes, chronic asthma, and intake of dietary supplements containing substances with antioxidant activity.

The study was approved by the Ethics Committee of the Hospital Regional Universitario de Malaga (Ref. 0255-N-22). It was performed in accordance with the Declaration of Helsinki principles and its subsequent amendments. The clinical and sociodemographic characteristics of the participants were assessed by the same group of investigators. Informed consent was obtained from all subjects participating in the study.

2.2. Stool Collection and Analysis

After four months following a GFD, participants were instructed to collect two stool samples on non-consecutive days, one on weekdays and the other during the weekend. Participants were provided with stool collection materials, including special plastic containers with crew caps labels, cold bags, isothermal boxes, and cold packs, and were instructed to collect at least 10 g of stool each time and to record the date and time of collection. All stool samples were stored in isothermal boxes with cold packs at 4–8 °C and sent to the laboratory within 48 h of collection. All samples were stored at −20 °C until they were processed. If any of these samples were positive, participants were asked to collect two new samples after 9 months of the CD diagnosis.

The concentration of GIPs in stool samples was measured using a lateral flow technique with the iVYCHECK GIP Stool kit (Biomedal S.L., Seville, Spain) based on the manufacturer's guidelines. This is a rapid immunochromatography test that detects GIPs in stool samples, with the possibility of a positive or negative result. This technique has demonstrated a sensitivity range of 95–100% and a specificity of 100% in several studies [26,27].

2.3. Anthropometric Measures

A scale and stadiometer (Seca 22, Hamburg, Germany) were employed to measure weight (kg) and height (m), respectively. Body mass index was calculated as (weight [Kg]/height [m^2]).

2.4. Dietary Assessment

A three-day record was employed to assess dietary intake. Participants received instructions from a trained dietitian to guarantee proper handling of the dietary. In addition, they received a photographic atlas with a chart of household measures and a list of portion sizes [28]. All of the meals consumed throughout the day were included in the survey, along with a detailed description of the food's quantity consumed (using the photographic atlas as a guide), its preparation (including cooking methods and sugar or fats added), and the brands of packaged foods consumed.

The Evalfinut 2.0 software, which includes the Spanish Food Composition Database [29], was used to analyze all diaries. The estimated energy (kilocalories) and macronutrient intake (measured in grams and including proteins, total fats, saturated fats, carbohydrates, simple sugar, and fiber), as well as the proportion of energy provided by each macronutrient, was calculated. Reference values for energy and nutrient consumption were drawn from the recommended energy mentioned previously and nutrient intake levels for the Spanish population [28]. The nutritional information on the labels of gluten-free products allowed us to determine the composition of these products.

Food was categorized using the NOVA categorization into four groups: unprocessed or minimally processed foods; processed culinary ingredients; processed foods; and ultra-processed foods [30]. It is the most widely used method for examining diets according to food processing and has been widely used by international agencies such as PAHO, WHO, and FAO [31–33].

In the event of a positive result in any of the samples delivered after 4 months of GFD, the team's dietitian made a phone call visit, which included a nutritional education session. During the visit, a review of the detailed revision of food and gluten-free products described in the three-day record was carried out, and the concern about any possible doubts about GFD and cross-contamination was addressed.

2.5. Statistical Analyses

The baseline characteristics of the study sample were described using descriptive statistics (mean standard deviation) for quantitative variables and the percentage of participants (%) for categorical variables. The Chi-square test was additionally used to explore differences in categorical variables.

A one-way analysis of covariance (ANOVA) after adjustment for age, sex, and BMI was employed to assess differences in food group consumption and NOVA food classification of children by fecal GIP detection (negative vs. positive). After controlling for age, sex, and BMI, ANOVA was used to assess dietary intakes by the percentage of energy consumed from UPF in children with CD (below 50% of daily energy intake vs. above 50% of daily calorie intake). The dietary intakes were compared by ANOVA after adjusting for age, sex, and BMI.

The Statistical Package for Social Sciences (IBM SPSS Statistics for Windows, Version 22. IBM Corp, Armonk, NY, USA) was used to analyze the data, and the statistical significance was set at $p < 0.05$.

3. Results

Characteristics of the study sample are displayed in Table 1. A total of 61 children with CD participated in the study (mean age 7.5 ± 3.9 years). More than half of the participants were norm weight (72%) and did not have other diseases (94%).

Table 1. Characteristics of the study participants (n = 61).

Variable	Mean (SD)
Age (years)	7.5 (3.9)
Sex (n [%])	
Male	24 (39.3)
Female	37 (60.7)
Weight (kg)	25.9 (13.3)
Height (m)	1.2 (0.2)
Body mass index categories (n [%])	
Underweight	2 (3.3)
Normoweight	44 (72.1)
Overweight	11 (18.0)
Obese	4 (6.6)
Energy (kcal) (n = 58)	1543.9 (462.2)
Fat (% of total energy intake)	38.2 (6.7)
Protein (% of total energy intake)	16.0 (4.0)
Carbohydrates (% of total energy intake)	44.2 (6.6)
NOVA food classification (n = 58)	
Unprocessed or minimally processed foods (kcal/day)	601.0 (215.8)
Unprocessed or minimally processed foods (%E)	39.8 (11.5)
Processed culinary ingredients (kcal/day)	102.3 (63.4)
Processed culinary ingredients (%E)	6.7 (3.4)
Processed Foods (kcal/day)	98.1 (84.1)
Processed Foods (%E)	6.2 (4.9)
Ultra-processed food and drink products (kcal)	739.4 (316.7)
Ultra-processed food and drink products (%Energy)	47.5 (13.1)
Fecal gluten immunogenic peptides (n [%]) (n = 60)	
Positive	8 (13.3)
Negative	52 (86.7)
Other diseases (yes, n [%])	4 (6.6)

Values shown as mean (standard deviation) unless otherwise indicated.

The percentage of participants with stool GIP detection according to months on a GFD are shown in Figure 1. After 4 months following a GFD, eight patients (13.3%) tested positive for stool GIP (GIP+), and 52 patients (86.7%) tested negative (GIP−). After 9 months following a GFD, one child remained GIP+. Specifically, GIPs were detected in the stools of 33% of children with CD before 2 years of age and of 13% and 10% of children diagnosed at 2–6 years and at an older age, 7–18 years, respectively (Figure 2).

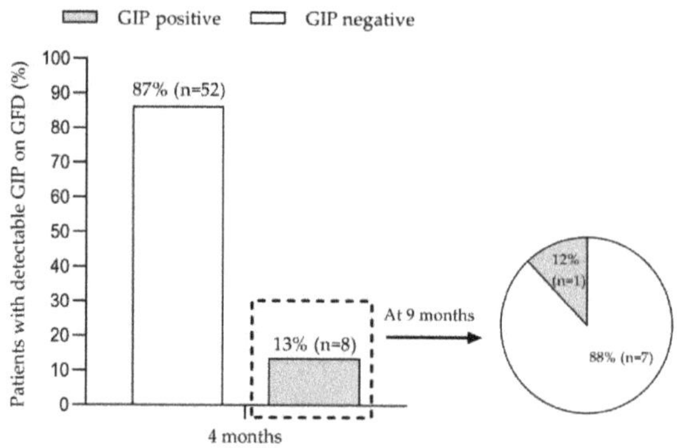

Figure 1. Stool gluten immunogenic peptide detection according to months following a gluten-free diet. GFD, gluten-free diet.

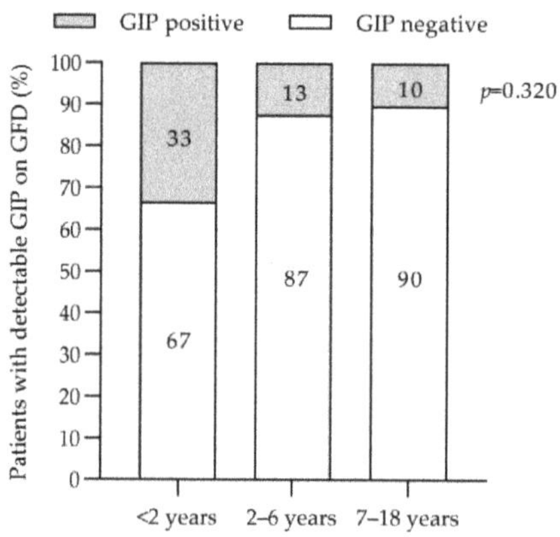

Figure 2. Stool gluten immunogenic peptide detection according to patient age. GIP, gluten immunogenic peptides. GFD, gluten-free diet.

The percentage of adequacy for energy, protein, and micronutrient profile intake by age group and sex according to Moreiras et al. [29] and other groups' recommendations [34] is shown in Figure 3. The adequacy for energy, fiber, and protein intake was 89%, 73%, and 189%, respectively. Regarding micronutrients, the adequacy for Vitamin D was 23%, the adequacy for folate was 53%, and the adequacy for calcium and magnesium was 62% and 57%, respectively. Furthermore, according to the recommendations by the European Food Safety Authority (EFSA) [35], the percentage of children that meet the carbohydrate and protein intake was 50% and 19%, respectively (Figure 4). A total of 66% of children exceed the recommended intake for fat. Additionally, all children (100%) exceeded the recommended intake for protein. No differences in dietary intake and NOVA food classification by fecal GIP detection (GIP− vs. GIP+) were found (Table 2) (all $p > 0.05$). There were no significant differences in the percentage of adequacy according to fecal GIP detection (GIP+ versus GIP−) ($p > 0.05$) (Supplementary Figure S1).

The percentage of adequacy for energy intake, fiber, protein, and micronutrients, recommended daily intake by a percentage of daily energy consumed from UPF in celiac children, is shown in Figure 5. The group with the highest intake of energy from UPF (above 50% of total energy) showed a lower intake of vitamin A ($p = 0.009$), calcium ($p = 0.027$), potassium ($p = 0.023$), and magnesium ($p = 0.046$) after adjusting the model for age, sex, and BMI.

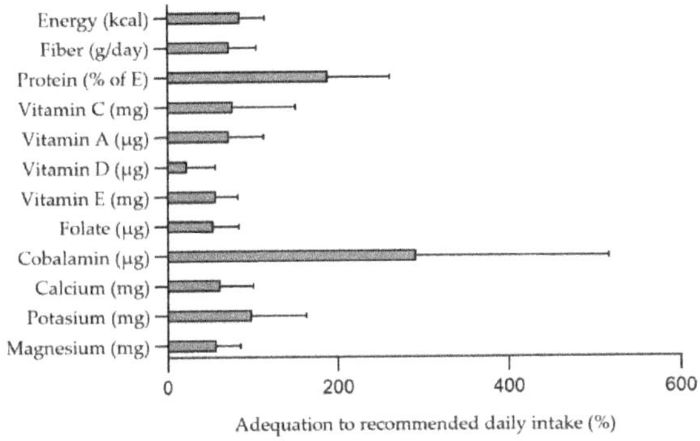

Figure 3. Percentage of adequacy for energy intake, fiber, protein, and micronutrients, recommended daily intake in children with celiac disease (n = 58).

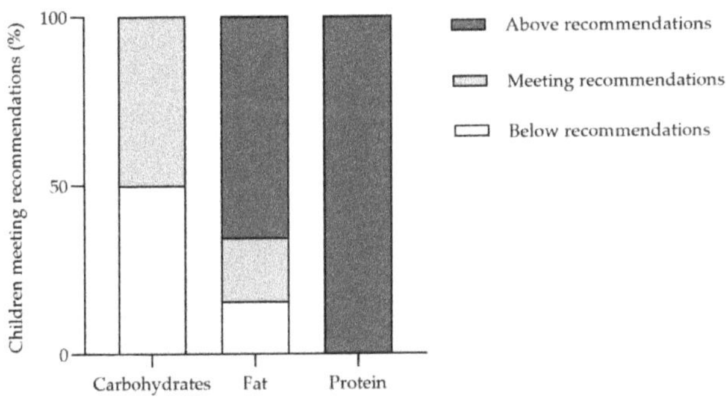

Figure 4. Children meeting European Food Safe Authority recommendations for carbohydrates, fat, and protein daily intakes.

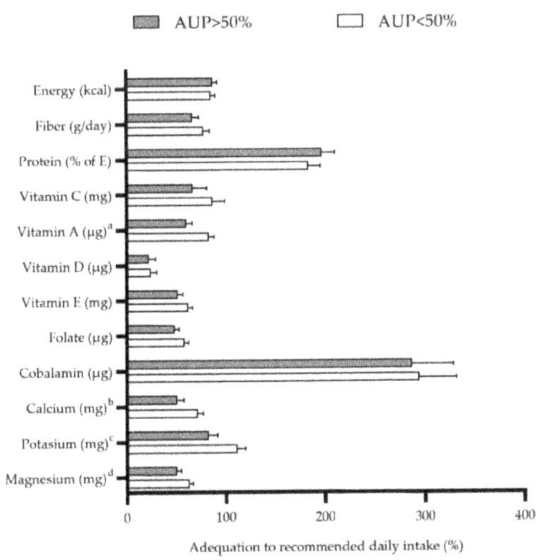

Figure 5. Percentage of adequacy for energy intake, fiber, protein, and micronutrients, recommended daily intake in children with celiac disease according to percentage of energy intake from ultra-processed food (n = 58). Values are shown as mean (standard error). Model is adjusted for age, sex, and body mass index (BMI). ^{a} $p = 0.009$; ^{b} $p = 0.027$; ^{c} $p = 0.023$; ^{d} $p = 0.046$.

Table 2. Differences in dietary intake by fecal gluten immunogenic peptide detection (negative vs. positive).

	Negative (n = 49)	Positive (n = 8)	p [a]	p [b]
Dietary intake				
Energy (kcal)	1559.3 (65.1)	1568.4 (161.1)	0.958	0.446
Fat (% of E)	38.9 (0.7)	38.7 (1.8)	0.929	0.953
Protein (% of E)	16.1 (0.6)	15.3 (1.4)	0.620	0.690
Carbohydrates (% E)	43.9 (0.9)	45.1 (2.4)	0.669	0.649
Fiber (g/day)	10.5 (0.7)	9.6 (1.7)	0.609	0.933
Sugar (g/day)	22.4 (2.0)	16.8 (5.2)	0.342	0.525
Vitamin A (µg)	320.2 (19.0)	274.6 (47.1)	0.373	0.493
Vitamin D (µg)	3.8 (0.7)	2.2 (1.8)	0.435	0.564
Vitamin E	4.4 (0.3)	5.2 (0.7)	0.380	0.234
Riboflavin (mg)	0.9 (0.05)	1.1 (0.1)	0.291	0.395
Folate (µg)	97.4 (6.3)	99.3 (15.5)	0.911	0.747
Cobalamin (µg)	4.2 (0.5)	3.3 (1.1)	0.511	0.609
Calcium (mg)	500.4 (38.5)	605.2 (95.4)	0.313	0.339
Vitamin C (mg)	46.1 (6.2)	31.8 (15.3)	0.390	0.721
Potasium (mg)	1496.8 (88.8)	1569.2 (219.7)	0.761	0.582
Magnesium (mg)	119.4 (6.7)	129.5 (16.5)	0.572	0.421
NOVA food classification				
Unprocessed or minimally processed foods (%E)	39.3 (1.7)	42.5 (4.1)	0.472	0.447
Processed culinary ingredients (%E)	6.7 (0.5)	7.6 (1.2)	0.489	0.463
Processed Foods (%E)	5.8 (0.7)	7.6 (1.7)	0.335	0.285
Ultra-processed food and drink products (%Energy)	48.6 (1.9)	41.3 (4.6)	0.146	0.088

[a] Model unadjusted [b] Model adjusted for age, sex, and body mass index. D, day; S, servings; W, week.

4. Discussion

We present, to our knowledge, the first study that evaluates adherence to the GFD in newly diagnosed patients with CD (<6 months). Our results suggest that early follow-up of the newly diagnosed CD is essential, both to assess adherence to the GFD, which is the only treatment currently available for the disease and to determine the GFD nutritional adequacy. It is unclear which is the most effective method to assess adherence to the GFD, and in this regard, our study demonstrates the role of stool GIP determination in the early monitoring of the GFD. On the other hand, it emphasizes the importance of nutritional intervention in the follow-up of these patients, as it has been shown that many patients with CD on GFD have nutritional imbalances and macronutrient and micronutrient deficits.

Adherence to the GFD is essential for mucosal recovery in newly diagnosed patients with CD. Non-adherence to the gluten-free diet can be due to different reasons. One of them may be due to the change in eating behaviour that occurs in the patient who changes his habits towards a GFD. Previous studies [36,37] have shown that a GFD leads to a higher intake of fat, protein, and UPF, although it has not yet been established whether nutritional imbalances have an impact on adherence to the GFD. In our cohort, there was no difference between patients with GIP+ and those with GIP−, suggesting that adherence is not influenced by dietary fat and protein intake, which is a common problem at the start of the diet. Determination of GIP in stool is a non-invasive method that provides direct information on recent gluten exposure [9]. In our study, we have assessed adherence to the GFD by determining GIP excreted in stool in a cohort of children with newly diagnosed CD. To identify intermittent gluten intakes, we carried out double determinations 4 months after CD diagnosis, indirectly analyzing the weekend diet and the weekday's diet, thus allowing the situation to be like what happens in real life. Ruiz-Carnicer et al. [3] and Stefanolo et al. [20] have already described the importance of multiple determinations to increase the sensitivity and specificity of the detection of GIPs in urine and stool, respectively. Our study reveals poor dietary compliance rates of 14% at 4 months, based on stool GIPs. Gerasimidis et al. [26] found 16% positive stool GIP in pediatric celiac patients who reported good GFD compliance after 6 months of GFD, while Comino et al. [19] demonstrated a stool

GIP positivity of 23% in celiac children after 6 months of GFD. Fernandez et al. [38] found 92.5% GFD adherence as determined by stool GIPs, with a large percentage of patients with positive stool GIPs but negative serological controls (anti-transglutaminase antibodies); in this study, lower GFD adherence was reported with increasing patient age and time since diagnosis of CD. Other authors have also described a worsening of adherence with longer disease progression [39]. In the long term, several aspects have been identified as the factors influencing this poor adherence to the GFD, such as less parental supervision (greater autonomy of patients, especially adolescents, who also eat more likely outside the home [19,40]), less awareness of the disease as symptomatology improves with adequate initial GFD adherence, and in some cases, the psychological overload of following a strict diet [19], especially in adolescents and young adults. In newly diagnosed celiac patients, especially in the pediatric population, these aspects should not be present, thus there is the need to emphasize appropriate nutritional counselling for patients and their families at the time of diagnosis, clear any doubts that arise in the process, and ensure early follow-up of celiac children after CD diagnosis. Interestingly, our study has identified the age group with the highest percentage of poor adherence to the GFD based on the determination of stool GIPs (under 2 years of age), as opposed to previous studies [19], and this may contribute to the development of age-specific follow-up strategies.

The assessment of positive GIPs together with a dietary record concomitant with stool sample collection allows the development of dietary interventions aimed at improving GFD adherence. In this regard, close counselling by a dietitian can improve GFD adherence, as demonstrated by the determination of GIP in control stool at 9 months in patients who were initially GIP+. Our results showed that 88% of those did not perform properly. GFDs were compliers after a nutritional education session. Regarding the consumption of UPF, we did not found differences between patients with GIP+ vs. GIP−, so we can speculate that the consumption of UPF does not allow to distinguish patients who adequately follow the diet. In this regard, it is important to emphasize the importance of appropriate initial advice to patients and families, providing them with information on the variety of gluten-free products available, especially natural gluten-free foods.

A GFD should be a balanced diet, which allows for optimal growth and development of children with CD. Nutritional imbalances have been described in patients with CD on GFD, including micronutrients (magnesium, calcium, iron, zinc, B vitamins, vitamin D, and folic acid) and fiber deficiencies. In our study, we observed deficient intake of vitamin D (only 27% of patients have an adequate intake, a similar percentage to that described in other studies in celiac patients, both in the diet prior to CD diagnosis and in the GFD [22]), as well as folate, calcium, and magnesium. We have also verified an inadequate fiber intake (73% adequacy), in line with other studies in patients with CD [22,24,41]. These findings suggest that nutritional counselling should be a priority for these patients at the beginning of the GDF, and early follow-up is essential to detect deficiencies that need to be corrected. In addition, we have also reported macronutrient imbalances in patients on a GFD. In our study, 66% of patients exceeded the recommended fat intake, and all of them exceeded the recommended protein intake [35]. Furthermore, a high percentage of total daily energy intake came from UPF, with these foods being mostly consumed in the morning and afternoon snacks. Other studies [42] have already demonstrated this high consumption of UPF, which may be due to several factors: on the one hand, the lower cost of manufactured gluten-free products compared to naturally gluten-free foods; on the other hand, the greater palatability and aesthetic appeal of the manufactured gluten-free products, especially for children; furthermore, families' lack of awareness of the different options available at the start of the GFD [42,43]. In our cohort, patients who consumed more energy from UPF had poor diet quality, as previously described by our research group [42].

Excess protein and fat intake in the diet of these patients, as well as high UPF consumption, has been linked to the development of other long-term health problems. On the one hand, excess fat and protein intake may contribute to the development of overweight or obesity, resulting in additional problems. Kabbani et al. [44] described an increase in the BMI in celiac patients over the course of the disease, especially in patients with higher GFD adherence: 4.4% of patients with low weight at diagnosis developed overweight or obesity, 17% of patients with normal weight at diagnosis developed overweight or obesity, and 17.3% of patients with overweight at diagnosis became obese. In addition, higher UPF consumption has been associated with an increased risk of overweight, obesity, metabolic syndrome, dyslipidemia, functional gastrointestinal disorders (irritable bowel syndrome and functional dyspepsia), recurrent wheezing, and depression in adult patients [45] and alterations of the gut microbiota [46]. All these aspects mostly lead to a worsening of digestive symptoms as well as the quality of life of these patients. This is another reason why action protocols should focus, among others, on nutritional education, to improve the quality of life and health of patients in the long term.

5. Strengths and Limitations

There are several limitations that should be highlighted. Firstly, this is a cross-sectional pilot study with a relatively small sample size, so results must be interpreted with caution. However, we present the first study to assess adherence to the GFD at such an early stage. Secondly, another limitation of our study is the lack of a control group, which is difficult given the assessment of a specific type of diet in the group of patients with CD. Thirdly, there has been no follow-up of the cohort, so we have not been able to evaluate the diet quality in the medium and long term; however, the aim of our study was to assess early disbalances resulting from the implementation of the GFD. It would be advisable to take these limitations into account and to recruit a larger number of patients.

6. Conclusions

The findings of our study demonstrate the role of stool GIP determination in monitoring GFD adherence in the first months after CD diagnosis, which may be key in the early detection of patients with transgressions or inadvertent gluten intakes. This may allow the development of specific follow-up strategies based on the initial determination of GIPs, as well as clinical management protocols. More studies are needed to correlate GIP positivity with serology, as well as studies with a control group, to increase the validity of the results. On the other hand, early monitoring of the diet of patients with CD was able to detect important nutritional imbalances and deficiencies, thus guiding the dietary advice of our celiac patients more precisely to prevent future nutritional diseases. We believe that it is important to highlight the participation of dietitians in the management of the disease to guide the GFD.

Supplementary Materials: The following are available online at https://www.mdpi.com/article/10.3390/nu15071761/s1, Supplementary Figure S1: Percentage of adequacy for energy intake, fiber, protein, and micronutrients recommended daily intake in children with celiac disease according to fecal detectable gluten immunogenic peptides (n = 58). Values are shown as mean (standard error). Model is adjusted for age, sex, and body mass index.

Author Contributions: Conceptualization, R.M.-M. and V.M.N.-L.; methodology, R.M.-M. and M.H.-L.; validation, R.M.-M., M.F.-A. and T.N.; formal analysis, M.F.-A.; investigation, R.M.-M., M.J.-M. and M.H.-L.; resources, R.M.-M., V.M.N.-L. and T.N.; data curation, R.M.-M., M.J.-M. and M.H.-L.; writing—original draft preparation, R.M.-M., M.J.-M., M.H.-L., M.F.-A., V.M.N.-L. and T.N.; writing—review and editing, R.M.-M., M.J.-M., M.H.-L., M.F.-A., V.M.N.-L. and T.N.; project administration, R.M.-M. and V.M.N.-L. funding acquisition, R.M.-M. and T.N. All authors have read and agreed to the published version of the manuscript.

Funding: This research was funded by the FEDER/Junta de Andalucía-Consejería de Transformación Económica, Industria, Conocimiento y Universidades/ Project No B-AGR-658. It was also partially funded with the grant "Investigation grant program by the Association of Celiacs and Sensitive to Gluten of the Community of Madrid". It also was partially funded by BIOMEDAL S.L.

Institutional Review Board Statement: The study was conducted in accordance with the Declaration of Helsinki and approved by the Ethics Committee of the Hospital Regional Universitario of Málaga, Spain (code: 0255-N-22).

Informed Consent Statement: Informed consent was obtained from all subjects involved in the study.

Data Availability Statement: The data presented in this study are available on request from the corresponding author.

Conflicts of Interest: The authors declare no conflict of interest. The funders had no role in the design of the study; in the collection, analyses, or interpretation of data; in the writing of the manuscript, or in the decision to publish the results.

References

1. Schuppan, D. Current Concepts of Celiac Disease Pathogenesis. *Gastroenterology* **2000**, *119*, 234–242. [CrossRef]
2. Caio, G.; Volta, U.; Sapone, A.; Leffler, D.A.; de Giorgio, R.; Catassi, C.; Fasano, A. Celiac Disease: A Comprehensive Current Review. *BMC Med.* **2019**, *17*, 142. [CrossRef]
3. Ruiz-Carnicer, A.; Garzon-Benavides, M.; Fombuena, B.; Segura, V.; Garcia-Fernandez, F.; Sobrino-Rodriguez, S.; Gomez-Izquierdo, L.; Montes-Cano, M.A.; Rodriguez-Herrera, A.; Millan, R.; et al. Negative Predictive Value of the Repeated Absence of Gluten Immunogenic Peptides in the Urisne of Treated Celiac Patients in Predicting Mucosal Healing: New Proposals for Follow-up in Celiac Disease. *Am. J. Clin. Nutr.* **2020**, *112*, 1240–1251. [CrossRef] [PubMed]
4. Singh, P.; Arora, A.; Strand, T.A.; Leffler, D.A.; Catassi, C.; Green, P.H.; Kelly, C.P.; Ahuja, V.; Makharia, G.K. Global Prevalence of Celiac Disease: Systematic Review and Meta-Analysis. *Clin. Gastroenterol. Hepatol.* **2018**, *16*, 823–836.e2. [CrossRef] [PubMed]
5. King, J.A.; Jeong, J.; Underwood, F.E.; Quan, J.; Panaccione, N.; Windsor, J.W.; Coward, S.; Debruyn, J.; Ronksley, P.E.; Shaheen, A.A.; et al. Incidence of Celiac Disease Is Increasing Over Time: A Systematic Review and Meta-Analysis. *Am. J. Gastroenterol.* **2020**, *115*, 507–525. [CrossRef]
6. Coto, L.; Sousa, C.; Cebolla, A. Individual Variability in Patterns and Dynamics of Fecal Gluten Immunogenic Peptides Excretion after Low Gluten Intake. *Eur. J. Nutr.* **2022**, *61*, 2033–2049. [CrossRef] [PubMed]
7. Myléus, A.; Reilly, N.R.; Green, P.H.R. Rate, Risk Factors, and Outcomes of Nonadherence in Pediatric Patients with Celiac Disease: A Systematic Review. *Clin. Gastroenterol. Hepatol.* **2020**, *18*, 562–573. [CrossRef]
8. Muhammad, H.; Reeves, S.; Jeanes, Y.M. Identifying and Improving Adherence to the Gluten-Free Diet in People with Coeliac Disease. *Proc. Nutr. Soc.* **2019**, *78*, 418–425. [CrossRef]
9. Volta, U.; Caio, G.; Stanghellini, V.; de Giorgio, R. The Changing Clinical Profile of Celiac Disease: A 15-Year Experience (1998–2012) in an Italian Referral Center. *BMC Gastroenterol.* **2014**, *14*, 194. [CrossRef]
10. El Péptido del Gluten en Heces Puede Ser Útil en el Seguimiento de la Enfermedad Celíaca—Evidencias en Pediatría. Available online: https://evidenciasenpediatria.es/articulo/7328/el-peptido-del-gluten-en-heces-puede-ser-util-en-el-seguimiento-de-la-enfermedad-celiaca?id=7328&titulo=el-peptido-del-gluten-en-heces-puede-ser-util-en-el-seguimiento-de-la-enfermedad-celiaca (accessed on 8 February 2023).
11. Husby, S.; Koletzko, S.; Korponay-Szabó, I.; Kurppa, K.; Mearin, M.L.; Ribes-Koninckx, C.; Shamir, R.; Troncone, R.; Auricchio, R.; Castillejo, G.; et al. European Society Paediatric Gastroenterology, Hepatology and Nutrition Guidelines for Diagnosing Coeliac Disease 2020. *J. Pediatr. Gastroenterol. Nutr.* **2020**, *70*, 141–156. [CrossRef]
12. Silvester, J.A.; Kurada, S.; Szwajcer, A.; Kelly, C.P.; Leffler, D.A.; Duerksen, D.R. Tests for Serum Transglutaminase and Endomysial Antibodies Do Not Detect Most Patients with Celiac Disease and Persistent Villous Atrophy on Gluten-Free Diets: A Meta-Analysis. *Gastroenterology* **2017**, *153*, 689. [CrossRef] [PubMed]
13. Comino, I.; Real, A.; Vivas, S.; Síglez, M.Á.; Caminero, A.; Nistal, E.; Casqueiro, J.; Rodríguez-Herrera, A.; Cebolla, Á.; Sousa, C. Monitoring of Gluten-Free Diet Compliance in Celiac Patients by Assessment of Gliadin 33-Mer Equivalent Epitopes in Feces. *Am. J. Clin. Nutr.* **2012**, *95*, 670–677. [CrossRef] [PubMed]
14. Laserna-Mendieta, E.J.; Casanova, M.J.; Arias, Á.; Arias-González, L.; Majano, P.; Mate, L.A.; Gordillo-Vélez, C.H.; Jiménez, M.; Angueira, T.; Tébar-Romero, E.; et al. Poor Sensitivity of Fecal Gluten Immunogenic Peptides and Serum Antibodies to Detect Duodenal Mucosal Damage in Celiac Disease Monitoring. *Nutrients* **2020**, *13*, 98. [CrossRef] [PubMed]
15. Syage, J.A.; Kelly, C.P.; Dickason, M.A.; Ramirez, A.C.; Leon, F.; Dominguez, R.; Sealey-Voyksner, J.A. Determination of Gluten Consumption in Celiac Disease Patients on a Gluten-Free Diet. *Am. J. Clin. Nutr.* **2018**, *107*, 201–207. [CrossRef] [PubMed]
16. Silvester, J.A.; Comino, I.; Kelly, C.P.; Sousa, C.; Duerksen, D.R.; Bernstein, C.N.; Cebolla, A.; Comino, I.; Dominguez, M.R.; Duerksen, D.R.; et al. Most Patients with Celiac Disease on Gluten-Free Diets Consume Measurable Amounts of Gluten. *Gastroenterology* **2020**, *158*, 1497–1499.e1. [CrossRef] [PubMed]
17. Moreno, M.D.L.; Sánchez-Muñoz, D.; Sanders, D.; Rodríguez-Herrera, A.; Sousa, C. Verifying Diagnosis of Refractory Celiac Disease with Urine Gluten Immunogenic Peptides as Biomarker. *Front. Med.* **2021**, *7*, 601854. [CrossRef]
18. Moreno, M.D.L.; Cebolla, Á.; Munõz-Suano, A.; Carrillo-Carrion, C.; Comino, I.; Pizarro, Á.; León, F.; Rodríguez-Herrera, A.; Sousa, C. Detection of Gluten Immunogenic Peptides in the Urine of Patients with Coeliac Disease Reveals Transgressions in the Gluten-Free Diet and Incomplete Mucosal Healing. *Gut* **2017**, *66*, 250–257. [CrossRef]

19. Comino, I.; Segura, V.; Ortigosa, L.; Espín, B.; Castillejo, G.; Garrote, J.A.; Sierra, C.; Millán, A.; Ribes-Koninckx, C.; Román, E.; et al. Prospective Longitudinal Study: Use of Faecal Gluten Immunogenic Peptides to Monitor Children Diagnosed with Coeliac Disease during Transition to a Gluten-Free Diet. *Aliment. Pharmacol. Ther.* **2019**, *49*, 1484–1492. [CrossRef]
20. Stefanolo, J.P.; Tálamo, M.; Dodds, S.; de la Paz Temprano, M.; Costa, A.F.; Moreno, M.L.; Pinto-Sánchez, M.I.; Smecuol, E.; Vázquez, H.; Gonzalez, A.; et al. Real-World Gluten Exposure in Patients with Celiac Disease on Gluten-Free Diets, Determined From Gliadin Immunogenic Peptides in Urine and Fecal Samples. *Clin. Gastroenterol. Hepatol.* **2021**, *19*, 484–491.e1. [CrossRef]
21. Coto, L.; Mendia, I.; Sousa, C.; Bai, J.C.; Cebolla, A. Determination of Gluten Immunogenic Peptides for the Management of the Treatment Adherence of Celiac Disease: A Systematic Review. *World J. Gastroenterol.* **2021**, *27*, 6306–6321. [CrossRef]
22. Salazar Quero, J.C.; Espín Jaime, B.; Rodríguez Martínez, A.; Argüelles Martín, F.; García Jiménez, R.; Rubio Murillo, M.; Pizarro Martín, A. Valoración Nutricional de La Dieta Sin Gluten. ¿Es La Dieta Sin Gluten Deficitaria En Algún Nutriente? *An. Pediatr.* **2015**, *83*, 33–39. [CrossRef]
23. di Nardo, G.; Villa, M.P.; Conti, L.; Ranucci, G.; Pacchiarotti, C.; Principessa, L.; Raucci, U.; Parisi, P. Nutritional Deficiencies in Children with Celiac Disease Resulting from a Gluten-Free Diet: A Systematic Review. *Nutrients* **2019**, *11*, 1588. [CrossRef]
24. Babio, N.; Alcázar, M.; Castillejo, G.; Recasens, M.; Martínez-Cerezo, F.; Gutiérrez-Pensado, V.; Masip, G.; Vaqué, C.; Vila-Martí, A.; Torres-Moreno, M.; et al. Patients with Celiac Disease Reported Higher Consumption of Added Sugar and Total Fat Than Healthy Individuals. *J. Pediatr. Gastroenterol. Nutr.* **2017**, *64*, 63–69. [CrossRef] [PubMed]
25. Zuccotti, G.; Fabiano, V.; Dilillo, D.; Picca, M.; Cravidi, C.; Brambilla, P. Intakes of Nutrients in Italian Children with Celiac Disease and the Role of Commercially Available Gluten-Free Products. *J. Hum. Nutr. Diet* **2013**, *26*, 436–444. [CrossRef]
26. Gerasimidis, K.; Zafeiropoulou, K.; Mackinder, M.; Ijaz, U.Z.; Duncan, H.; Buchanan, E.; Cardigan, T.; Edwards, C.A.; McGrogan, P.; Russell, R.K. Comparison of Clinical Methods with the Faecal Gluten Immunogenic Peptide to Assess Gluten Intake in Coeliac Disease. *J. Pediatr. Gastroenterol. Nutr.* **2018**, *67*, 356–360. [CrossRef]
27. Roca, M.; Donat, E.; Masip, E.; Crespo-Escobar, P.; Fornes-Ferrer, V.; Polo, B.; Ribes-Koninckx, C. Detection and Quantification of Gluten Immunogenic Peptides in Feces of Infants and Their Relationship with Diet. *Rev. Esp. Enferm. Dig.* **2019**, *111*, 106–110. [CrossRef] [PubMed]
28. Guía Para Estudios Dietéticos. Albúm Fotográfico de Alimentos—Universidad de Granada. Available online: https://editorial.ugr.es/libro/guia-para-estudios-dieteticos_137495/ (accessed on 10 February 2023).
29. Moreiras, O.; Carbajal, Á.; Cabrera, L.; Cuadrado, C. *Tablas de Composición de Alimentos*; Pirámide: Madrid, Spain, 2018; p. 496.
30. Moubarac, J.C.; Batal, M.; Louzada, M.L.; Martinez Steele, E.; Monteiro, C.A. Consumption of Ultra-Processed Foods Predicts Diet Quality in Canada. *Appetite* **2017**, *108*, 512–520. [CrossRef]
31. OPS. *Alimentos y Bebidas Ultraprocesados en América Latina: Tendencias, Efecto Sobre la Obesidad e Implicaciones Para las Políticas Públicas*; Departamento de Enfermedades no Transmisibles y Salud Mental: Washington, DC, USA, 2015; p. 76.
32. FAO. *Guidelines on the Collection of Information on Food Processing through Food Consumption Surveys*; FAO: Rome, Italy, 2015.
33. Monteiro, C.A.; Moubarac, J.C.; Cannon, G.; Ng, S.W.; Popkin, B. Ultra-Processed Products Are Becoming Dominant in the Global Food System. *Obes. Rev.* **2013**, *14* (Suppl. S2), 21–28. [CrossRef] [PubMed]
34. Madrigal, C.; Soto-Méndez, M.J.; Hernández-Ruiz, Á.; Valero, T.; Ávila, J.M.; Ruiz, E.; Villoslada, F.L.; Leis, R.; de Victoria, E.M.; Moreno, J.M.; et al. Energy Intake, Macronutrient Profile and Food Sources of Spanish Children Aged One To. *Nutrients* **2020**, *12*, 893. [CrossRef]
35. Dietary Reference Values | EFSA. Available online: https://www.efsa.europa.eu/en/topics/topic/dietary-reference-values (accessed on 10 February 2023).
36. Ferrara, P.; Cicala, M.; Tiberi, E.; Spadaccio, C.; Marcella, L.; Gatto, A.; Calzolari, P.; Castellucci, G. High Fat Consumption in Children with Celiac Disease. *Acta Gastroenterol. Belg.* **2009**, *72*, 296–300.
37. Forchielli, M.L.; Diani, L.; Labriola, F.; Bolasco, G.; Rocca, A.; Salfi, N.C.; Leone, A.; Miserocchi, C.; Andreozzi, L.; Levi Della Vida, F.; et al. Gluten Deprivation: What Nutritional Changes Are Found During the First Year in Newly Diagnosed Coeliac Children? *Nutrients* **2019**, *12*, 60. [CrossRef]
38. Fernández Miaja, M.; Díaz Martín, J.J.; Jiménez Treviño, S.; Suárez González, M.; Bousoño García, C. Estudio de La Adherencia a La Dieta Sin Gluten En Pacientes Celiacos. *An. Pediatr.* **2021**, *94*, 377–384. [CrossRef]
39. Al Sarkhy, A.; El Mouzan, M.I.; Saeed, E.; Alanazi, A.; Alghamdi, S.; Anil, S.; Assiri, A. Clinical Characteristics of Celiac Disease and Dietary Adherence to Gluten-Free Diet among Saudi Children. *Pediatr. Gastroenterol. Hepatol. Nutr.* **2015**, *18*, 23–29. [CrossRef] [PubMed]
40. Comino, I.; Fernández-Bañares, F.; Esteve, M.; Ortigosa, L.; Castillejo, G.; Fambuena, B.; Ribes-Koninckx, C.; Sierra, C.; Rodríguez-Herrera, A.; Salazar, J.C.; et al. Fecal Gluten Peptides Reveal Limitations of Serological Tests and Food Questionnaires for Monitoring Gluten-Free Diet in Celiac Disease Patients. *Am. J. Gastroenterol.* **2016**, *111*, 1456. [CrossRef] [PubMed]
41. Shepherd, S.J.; Gibson, P.R. Nutritional Inadequacies of the Gluten-Free Diet in Both Recently-Diagnosed and Long-Term Patients with Coeliac Disease. *J. Hum. Nutr. Diet.* **2013**, *26*, 349–358. [CrossRef] [PubMed]
42. Nestares, T.; Martín-Masot, R.; Flor-Alemany, M.; Bonavita, A.; Maldonado, J.; Aparicio, V.A. Influence of Ultra-Processed Foods Consumption on Redox Status and Inflammatory Signaling in Young Celiac Patients. *Nutrients* **2021**, *13*, 156. [CrossRef]
43. Penagini, F.; Dilillo, D.; Meneghin, F.; Mameli, C.; Fabiano, V.; Zuccotti, G.V. Gluten-Free Diet in Children: An Approach to a Nutritionally Adequate and Balanced Diet. *Nutrients* **2013**, *5*, 4553–4565. [CrossRef]

44. Kabbani, T.A.; Goldberg, A.; Kelly, C.P.; Pallav, K.; Tariq, S.; Peer, A.; Hansen, J.; Dennis, M.; Leffler, D.A. Body Mass Index and the Risk of Obesity in Coeliac Disease Treated with the Gluten-Free Diet. *Aliment. Pharmacol. Ther.* **2012**, *35*, 723–729. [CrossRef]
45. Lane, M.M.; Davis, J.A.; Beattie, S.; Gómez-Donoso, C.; Loughman, A.; O'Neil, A.; Jacka, F.; Berk, M.; Page, R.; Marx, W.; et al. Ultraprocessed Food and Chronic Noncommunicable Diseases: A Systematic Review and Meta-Analysis of 43 Observational Studies. *Obes. Rev.* **2021**, *22*, e13146. [CrossRef]
46. Aguayo-Patrón, S.V.; Calderón de la Barca, A.M. Old Fashioned vs. Ultra-Processed-Based Current Diets: Possible Implication in the Increased Susceptibility to Type 1 Diabetes and Celiac Disease in Childhood. *Foods* **2017**, *6*, 100. [CrossRef]

nutrients

MDPI

Article

Nutritional Composition of Breakfast in Children and Adolescents with and without Celiac Disease in Spain—Role of Gluten-Free Commercial Products

Natalia Úbeda †, María Purificación González *, María Achón , Ángela García-González , Catalina Ballestero-Fernández, Violeta Fajardo and Elena Alonso-Aperte †

Departamento de Ciencias Farmacéuticas y de la Salud, Facultad de Farmacia, Universidad San Pablo-CEU, CEU Universities, Urbanización Montepríncipe, Boadilla del Monte, 28660 Madrid, Spain; nubeda@ceu.es (N.Ú.); achontu@ceu.es (M.A.); angargon@ceu.es (Á.G.-G.); catalinaballestero@gmail.com (C.B.-F.); violeta.fajardomartin@ceu.es (V.F.); eaperte@ceu.es (E.A.-A.)

* Correspondence: mpgonzal@ceu.es; Tel.: +34-913724719

† These authors share senior authorship.

Abstract: Eating a nutritionally balanced breakfast can be a challenge when following a gluten-free diet (GFD). We assessed the ingredients and nutrient composition of 364 gluten-free breakfast products (GFPs) and 348 gluten-containing counterparts (GCCs), and we analysed the nutritional quality of breakfast in a group of Spanish children and adolescents with celiac disease (CD) (n = 70), as compared to controls (n = 67). Food intakes were estimated using three 24 h dietary records. The composition of GFPs and GCCs was retrieved from the package labels of commercially available products. Most participants (98.5%) ate breakfast daily, and only one person in each group skipped breakfast once. The breakfast contribution of the total daily energy was 19% in participants with CD and 20% in controls. CD patients managed a balanced breakfast in terms of energy (54% from carbohydrates; 12% from proteins; 34% from lipids) and key food groups (cereals, dairy, fruits), but their intake of fruits needs improvement. Compared to controls, breakfast in the CD group provided less protein and saturated fat, a similar amount of carbohydrates and fibre, and more salt. Fibre is frequently added to GFPs, but these contain less protein because of the flours used in formulation. Gluten-free bread contains more fat and is more saturated than is GCC. Sugars, sweets, and confectionery contribute more to energy and nutrient intakes in participants with CD, while grain products do so in controls. Overall, breakfast on a GFD can be adequate, but can be improved by GFPs reformulation and a lower consumption of processed foods.

Keywords: breakfast; children; adolescents; gluten-free

1. Introduction

Breakfast is identified as a significant contributor to a healthy lifestyle and represents an important source of key nutrients in the diet of children and adolescents [1]. However, there is still no unanimous consensus on whether breakfast is the most important meal of the day [2–4]. Spanish dietary recommendations suggest that a healthy and a nutrient density-adequate breakfast should contribute around 20–25% of the total daily energy intake and it should constitute the triad: (1) dairy products (a glass of milk, fresh yogurt, or a portion of cheese); (2) cereals (bread, cookies, homemade pastries, or breakfast cereals); and (3) fruit or natural juice. Furthermore, it could also be complemented on some occasions by other protein foods, such as eggs, ham, nuts, etc. [2,5].

According to results by Ruiz et al. [2] from the Anthropometry, Intake and Energy Balance (ANIBES) Study in Spain, children consume breakfast frequently (93.4%); however, the highest prevalence of irregular and non-breakfast consumers were clearly identified among adolescents (12.3% and 7.6%, respectively). Breakfast contributed between 17 and

18% of the total daily energy intake in these population groups. The most consumed breakfast food was chocolate (mainly as chocolate-flavoured milk and powder), followed by baked goods and pastries, whole milk, and semi-skimmed milk. Recently, similar results were found by Cuadrado-Soto et al. [1] from the National Dietary Survey on the Child and Adolescent Population (ENALIA) Study, also conducted in Spain. According to these studies, Spanish youth are not meeting recommendations for breakfast, a fact that poses the intriguing question of what may be happening when there is a food restriction in cereal consumption, as in the case of people with celiac disease (CD). Wheat and other gluten-containing cereals are very common in the Spanish diet, so taking a complete and nutritionally adequate breakfast can be a real challenge for children and adolescents with CD. If unmastered, the selection of suitable gluten-free foods for breakfast is difficult and expensive for celiacs, and may turn boring and exhausting, causing youngsters to skip breakfast.

Skipping breakfast is more frequent among women, later adolescents, those living in single-parent households, and in lower socioeconomic positions [6]. Breakfast skipping has also been found to be positively correlated with overweight/obesity (OW/OB) and biomarkers of metabolic diseases [6–10]. Particularly, the Food, Physical Activity, Child development and Obesity (ALADINO) and the Healthy Lifestyle in Europe by Nutrition in Adolescence (HELENA) Studies, carried out on Spanish children, confirm the association between not eating breakfast daily and a higher prevalence of OW/OB [11–13]. However, these results should be interpreted carefully since there are other studies which show contrary results [7,14].

The limited evidence from longitudinal studies among children/adolescents suggests that skipping breakfast is also related with higher fasting insulin levels and that daily breakfast practice is linked to a significantly lower homeostasis model assessment—insulin resistance (HOMA-IR) index [4,15]. Moreover, cognitive function could also be affected by eating an adequate breakfast. Its regular consumption was similarly correlated with better academic performance scores [16,17].

Many studies also confirm the impact of a healthy breakfast, showing higher daily nutrient intakes, an improved daily total nutrient intake, a better compliance with nutritional recommendations, and a better overall diet quality [18,19]. Specifically, children and adolescents who eat breakfast on a regular basis, compared to those who do not eat breakfast, consume higher amounts of energy, dietary fibre, fruits, and vegetables, and fewer sugar-sweetened beverages [4]. In this context, those who eat a daily breakfast consisting of dairy products, breakfast cereals, and fruits have higher daily intakes of some critical micronutrients for their age group (calcium, iron, potassium, magnesium, zinc, and iodine) compared to breakfast skippers [4].

To our knowledge, there are no studies assessing breakfast in a population with CD. A strict and lifelong adherence to a gluten-free diet (GFD) is the first-line treatment and, currently, is the only effective therapy for patients with CD and all other gluten-related disorders, such as non-celiac gluten sensitivity or wheat allergy [20].

CD is a major public health problem worldwide, with the following global prevalence data depending on the diagnostic method employed: 1.4% based on serologic tests and 0.7% according to biopsy [21,22]. The prevalence of CD varies with sex, age, and geographic region. Particularly, different studies show that the incidence rates of CD in children are significantly higher (0.9% vs. 0.5%) than in adults [21,23–25]. In Spain, current CD prevalence in children could be much greater than that monitored in other European countries [24]. Diagnoses of the early stages of CD and the life-long exclusion of gluten are the main therapeutic approaches to the disease, which is multisystemic and affects multiple organs. Subjects with CD are more likely to have digestive problems because gluten triggers an immune response in the small intestine that impacts the mucosa and lowers the ability to absorb nutrients in the body. In children and adolescents with CD, malabsorption can cause growth and developmental problems such us weight loss, anaemia, irritability, short stature, delayed puberty, tooth enamel defects, neurological symptoms, including attention-deficit/hyperactivity disorder, learning disabilities, headaches, chronic fatigue and, over time, osteoporosis [26].

Due to the limitations of a GFD, children and adolescents particularly consume many processed products made specifically for them [27]. According to some authors, abusive use of these products can have long-term consequences, including systemic inflammation or intestinal microbiota alteration, that appear to contribute to the persistence of nutritional deficiencies [28] and cardiometabolic-related pathologies, such as obesity [29,30] or cardiovascular disease [31]. Because of cultural dietary habits and food recommendations for breakfast, breakfast is the meal of the day in which gluten-free processed foods are more likely to be introduced in Spain.

Taken together, all the aforementioned studies warrant the importance of studying breakfast habits to prevent serious health issues. There is very limited information on children and adolescents with CD, especially with regard to their breakfast diet. Therefore, the present study firstly aimed to assess the nutritional quality (based on ingredients and nutrients) of processed cereal-based products commonly consumed at breakfast, e.g., breads, breakfast cereals, bakery products, etc., both gluten-free (GFPs) and their gluten-containing counterparts (GCCs). Furthermore, the second objective was to analyse the breakfast quality (all foods included) of a group of Spanish children and adolescents with CD compared to a group of similar age and gender characteristics without the disease (control). This analysis was based on the evaluation of the consumption of the different food groups recommended by the Spanish Society of Community Nutrition (Sociedad Española de Nutrición Comunitaria, SENC) [5] (dairy products, cereals, fruits, etc.) as well as the quality of their nutritional composition. Processed foods are generally recognised as a source of high energy, saturated fats, trans-fatty acids, sugar, and salt. An excessive intake of these nutrients is perceived as the main risk reason for developing some of the major public health problems such as OW/OB, type II diabetes, cancer, and cardiovascular diseases [32]. Results should be valuable for nutritional education and food reformulation, especially when developing strategies to improve nutritional quality and reduce the consumption of processed GFPs for breakfast.

2. Participants and Methods

2.1. Participants

Current dietary data were obtained in a cross-sectional survey in children and adolescents diagnosed with celiac disease (CD) and healthy controls. The Celiac and Gluten Sensitive Association (Asociación de Celiacos y Sensibles al Gluten de Madrid, Spain) helped in the recruitment of the participants. The eligibility criteria for the CD group included ages between 4 and 18 years old, having a certified diagnosis of CD, being on a gluten-free diet (GFD) for more than a year, not consuming pharmacological supplements, and not being affected by digestive discomfort at the time of dietary assessment. Adherence to the GFD was tested in blood samples from all participants through the analysis of immunoglobulin A (IgA) antitissue transglutaminase antibodies (IgA-tTG). The control group (healthy) participants were enlisted from the general population when meeting the following inclusion criteria: healthy status (absence of diagnosed chronic disease); not having symptoms or signs of any digestive disease; and not taking pharmacological or nutritional supplements.

All subjects and guardians or caregivers were informed and asked for a written consent to participate before enrolling. The study was conducted following the legal requirements and guidelines for good clinical practice, as well as the World Medical Association Declaration of Helsinki on Ethical Principles for Medical Research involving Human Subjects (revised in October 2008). The procedure was authorised by the Ethics Committee for Human Studies in Universidad San Pablo-CEU (Authorization number 102–15).

2.2. *Ingredients and Nutrient Content of Breakfast Products*

The gluten-free products (GFPs) composition database, developed by our research team and available at the Universidad San Pablo-CEU institutional repository [33,34], was used for GFPs composition data. This food database was compiled using the nutritional composition and ingredient list data from labels, as previously described [34]. Gluten-containing counterparts (GCCs) were chosen from retail stores and were matched to GFPs based on the same product (equal name and presentation) and greatest similarity in ingredient list. Ingredient and nutrient data from GCCs were also collected from the labelling on their packaging. Nutritional compositional of GFPs, currently available on the market, was evaluated in contrast to their GCCs.

Ingredients were chosen according to their impact on the nutritional profile of GFPs and GCCs and because of their critical effects on human health (starchy ingredients, fats, sugars, and fibre). In particular, the top ten most frequently used ingredients were considered. To analyse the frequency of use of these critical ingredients in the formulation of GFPs and GCCs, the breakfast products were organised in the following groups: bread and similar; breakfast cereals, biscuits, sweets, and semi-sweets, pastries and cakes, and churros (a traditional Spanish breakfast food consisting of a deep-fried dough made up of wheat and modelled in long tubes).

2.3. *Food Habits and Nutrient Intakes*

Firstly, a trained dietitian collected diverse information from the participants (personal data, family history of disease, and medication) during a face-to-face interview. According to the recommendations of the European Food Safety Authority [35], an individual's diet was estimated by applying three 24 h dietary records. The dietitian completed the first record with the assistance of the volunteers' relatives when it was necessary. The other two 24 h dietary records were fulfilled via phone call with a time difference interval of one month. A Sunday or a holiday was recalled for one of the three 24 h dietary records. GFPs brands were registered and the composition of all GFPs consumed was included in the database of the software used for analysis. As we previously explained [36], labels do not record data on micronutrient composition; therefore, data on micronutrient intake from these products were not quantified.

The assessment of energy and nutrient intakes was carried out using the DIAL® software, version 3.15 (Alce Ingeniería, Madrid, Spain) [37].

2.4. *Statistical Analysis*

For data analysis, IBM SPSS® Statistics for Windows (version 27.0, Somers, NY, USA, 2021) was used. A Kolmogorov–Smirnov test was applied to confirm the normality of the target variables. Results are shown as mean ± standard deviation. Mean differences between GFPs and GCCs were assessed using the Student's *t*-test. The analysis of categorical variables (descriptive data on ingredients) was handled using chi-squared test, and data are reported as frequencies (number of foods including a specific ingredient) and percentages (based on the total products within the group). Statistical significance was regarded only when p-values were lower than 0.05.

3. Results

A total of 70 participants with celiac disease (CD) (50% females and 80% children) and 67 non-celiac (control) (39% females; 69% children) took part in the survey. Mean age was 10.1 ± 3.7 for participants with CD and 10.3 ± 3.5 for controls. Most participants (98.5%) consumed breakfast every day, and only one person in each group skipped breakfast once.

3.1. *Ingredients Used in Gluten-Free and Gluten-Containing Breakfast Products*

A total of 364 GFPs and 348 GCCs were evaluated for ingredient and nutrient composition. Tables 1 and 2 display the type of flours and starches used as ingredients in the formulation of GFPs and GCCs commonly consumed at breakfast by Spanish children and adolescents.

As expected, GFPs are made with gluten-free flours such as rice, maize, pseudocereal, and legume flours; however, GCCs are mainly composed of wheat, rye, oat, and barley flours, regardless of the product group. Corn and rice cereal flours are the most frequently used, followed by legume flours in GFPs, whereas they are rarely used in GCCs. Notably, the only whole meal flour used is wheat flour, and it is only found in GCCs such as bread and similar, breakfast cereals, biscuits, sweets, and semi-sweet products. Regarding starches, a statistically higher frequency of use is observed among GFPs (Table 2). Gluten-free bread and similar, biscuits, sweets, semi-sweets, pastries, and cakes mainly include starch from corn, rice, potato, and tapioca. Only corn and wheat starch are used in GCCs.

Table 3 includes fat ingredients used in the formulation of GFPs and GCCs. Sunflower oil is the most frequently used ingredient in all breakfast products studied, and gluten-free breads include this oil more frequently, compared to GCCs. The least often used fats are palm, cocoa, coconut, butter, and cream in all groups of breakfast products, with hardly any significant differences between GFPs and GCCs. Margarines made from palm, rapeseed, coconut, and sunflower are more frequently used in the formulation of GFPs, especially in the case of bread and similar, biscuits, sweets and semi-sweets, and pastries and cakes. Eighty five percent of gluten-free pastries and cakes include added emulsifiers, which are absent in GCCs. The frequent use of additives of a fatty nature in all the breakfast products studied, including bread, is remarkable, except for gluten-containing and gluten-free churros.

The types of sugars and sweeteners and the frequency of use in the formulation of GFPs and GCCs commonly consumed at breakfast is shown in Table 4. A significant number of all food groups consumed include a wide variety of sugars, particularly sucrose, dextrose, glucose, and fructose syrup. Except for churros and gluten-containing pastries and cakes, between 60 to 85% of sweet breakfast products contain added sucrose, both GFPs as well as GCCs. Sucrose addition to bread, both gluten-free and regular, is also frequent (45% of products). Dextrose is significantly more frequently used in gluten-free bread and similar, pastries and cakes, as compared to GCCs.

Table 5 includes the fibre-type ingredients used in GFPs and GCCs. Fibre is more frequently added to GFPs compared to GCCs, especially in the case of bread and similar and pastries and cakes. These breakfast products mainly include hydroxypropyl methyl cellulose, guar gum, and xanthan gum. In addition, psyllium and bamboo are found in the bread and similar group.

3.2. Energy and Nutrient Composition of Gluten-Free and Gluten-Containing Breakfast Products

Table 6 shows the average energy content and nutrient composition of foods typically consumed for breakfast among Spanish children and adolescents, i.e., bread, breakfast cereals, biscuits, bakery products, and churros. Only gluten-free breakfast cereals show no nutritional differences with their GCCs. However, gluten-free breads contain a higher amount of fat and saturated fat, sugars, fibre, and salt, and a lower amount of protein, compared to GCCs. Gluten-free biscuits provide a higher amount of carbohydrates and a lower amount of protein; gluten-free pastries and cakes provide less energy, sugars, and protein, but have increased fibre and salt contents. Finally, churros provide less protein and salt, as compared to GCCs.

Table 1. Types of flour and frequency of use in the formulation of gluten-free and gluten-containing products commonly consumed for breakfast.

Breakfast Product		n	Rice n (%)	Corn n (%)	Millet n (%)	Amaranth n (%)	Legumes n (%)	Nut n (%)	Wheat n (%)	Whole Meal Wheat n (%)	Rye n (%)	Barley n (%)	Malt n (%)	Oat n (%)	Linseed n (%)
Bread and similar	GFPs	100	62 (62.0) ***	21(21.0) ***	16 (16.5) **	1 (2.4)	10 (10.5) **	1 (1.0)	0 (0.0) ***	0 (0.0)	1 (1.0) ***	0 (0.0)	0 (0.0) ***	0 (0.0)	11 (11.3)
	GCCs	101	14 (14.0)	3 (3.0)	4 (4.0)	0 (0.0)	25 (24.8)	0 (0.0)	89 (88.1)	6 (5.9)	25 (24.8)	1 (0.0)	22 (21.8)	4 (4.0)	18 (17.8)
Breakfast cereals	GFPs	35	15 (42.9)	27 (77.1) *	0 (0.0)	3 (8.6)	1 (2.9)	3 (8.6)	0 (0.0) ***	0 (0.0) ***	0 (0.0)	0 (0.0)	1 (2.9) **	5 (14.3) *	1 (2.9)
	GCCs	30	10 (33.3)	14 (46.7)	0 (0.0)	0 (0.0)	0 (0.0)	0 (0.0)	12 (40.0)	11 (36.7)	0 (0.0)	3 (10.0)	9 (30.0)	11 (36.7)	0 (0.0)
Biscuits, sweets, and semi-sweets	GFPs	96	55 (57.3) ***	61(63.5) ***	0 (0.0)	0 (0.0)	24 (25.0) ***	0 (0.0)	0 (0.0) ***	0 (0.0) ***	0 (0.0)	0 (0.0)	0 (0.0)	0 (0.0)	0 (0.0)
	GCCs	95	8 (8.4)	3 (3.2)	0 (0.0)	0 (0.0)	2 (2.1)	0 (0.0)	95 (100.0)	16 (16.8)	0 (0.0)	0 (0.0)	5 (5.3)	0 (0.0)	0 (0.0)
Pastries and cakes	GFPs	127	48 (37.8) ***	17(13.4) ***	0 (0.0)	0 (0.0)	28 (22.0) ***	15(11.8) ***	0 (0.0) ***	0 (0.0)	1 (0.8)	0 (0.0)	0 (0.0)	0 (0.0) **	3 (2.4)
	GCCs	116	6 (5.2)	0 (0.0)	0 (0.0)	0 (0.0)	5 (4.3)	0 (0.0)	113 (97.4)	0 (0.0)	3 (2.6)	3 (2.6)	0 (0.0)	9 (7.8)	0 (0.0)
Churros	GFPs	6	0 (0.0)	0 (0.0)	0 (0.0)	0 (0.0)	0 (0.0)	0 (0.0)	0 (0.0) ***	0 (0.0)	0 (0.0)	0 (0.0)	0 (0.0)	0 (0.0)	0 (0.0)
	GCCs	6	0 (0.0)	0 (0.0)	0 (0.0)	0 (0.0)	1 (16.7)	0 (0.0)	6 (100.0)	0 (0.0)	0 (0.0)	0 (0.0)	0 (0.0)	0 (0.0)	0 (0.0)

Results are expressed as frequency (n) of products, including a specific ingredient, and percentage based on the total products within the group. * $p < 0.05$ ** $p < 0.01$ *** $p < 0.001$ gluten-free products (GFPs) vs. gluten-containing counterparts (GCCs) within the same food group. Legumes: legumes, carob. Malt: malt, barley malt, rye malt, and maize malt.

Table 2. Types of starch and frequency of use in the formulation of gluten-free and gluten-containing products commonly consumed for breakfast.

Breakfast Product		n	Corn n (%)	Rice n (%)	Potato n (%)	Tapioca n (%)	Modified n (%)	Wheat n (%)
Bread and similar	GFPs	100	91 (91.0) ***	28 (28.0) ***	7 (7.0) *	16 (16.0) ***	1 (1.0)	0 (0.0) *
	GCCs	101	11 (10.9)	0 (0.0)	1 (1.0)	2 (2.0)	1 (1.0)	6 (5.9)
Breakfast cereals	GFPs	35	0 (0.0)	0 (0.0)	0 (0.0)	0 (0.0)	0 (0.0)	0 (0.0)
	GCCs	30	1 (3.3)	0 (0.0)	0 (0.0)	0 (0.0)	1 (3.3)	1 (3.3)
Biscuits, sweets, and semi-sweets	GFPs	96	59 (61.5) ***	26 (27.1) ***	29 (30.2) ***	4 (4.2) *	0 (0.0)	0 (0.0) ***
	GCCs	95	1 (1.1)	1 (1.1)	0 (0.0)	0 (0.0)	0 (0.0)	13 (13.7)
Pastries and cakes	GFPs	127	108 (85.0) ***	29 (22.8) ***	27 (21.3) ***	12 (9.4) **	2 (1.6) *	1 (0.8)
	GCCs	116	10 (8.6)	0 (0.0)	3 (2.6)	0 (0.0)	8 (6.9)	5 (4.3)
Churros	GFPs	6	3 (50.0) *	0 (0.0)	0 (0.0)	0 (0.0)	0 (0.0)	0 (0.0)
	GCCs	6	0 (0.0)	0 (0.0)	0 (0.0)	0 (0.0)	0 (0.0)	0 (0.0)

Results are expressed as frequency (n) of products, including a specific ingredient, and percentage based on the total products within the group. * $p < 0.05$ ** $p < 0.01$ *** $p < 0.001$ gluten-free products (GFPs) vs. gluten-containing counterparts (GCCs) within the same food group.

Table 3. Types of fat and frequency of use in the formulation of gluten-free and gluten-containing products commonly consumed for breakfast.

Breakfast Product		*n*	Sunflower *n* (%)	Palm *n* (%)	Olive *n* (%)	Cocoa *n* (%)	Rapeseed Oil *n* (%)	Margarine 1 *n* (%)	Margarine 2 *n* (%)	Coconut Oil *n* (%)	Animal Fat *n* (%)	Emulsifiers *n* (%)
Bread and similar	GFPs	100	70 (70.0) **	5 (5.0)	13 (13.0)	1 (1.0)	7 (7.1)	1 (1.0)	29 (29.0) ***	27 (27.0) ***	0 (0.0)	59 (59.0)
	GCCs	101	49 (48.5)	4 (4.0)	10 (9.9)	1 (1.0)	3 (3.0)	1 (1.0)	2 (2.0)	4 (4.0)	1 (1.0)	51 (50.5)
Breakfast cereals	GFPs	35	10 (28.6)	4 (11.4)	0 (0.0)	12 (34.3) *	1 (2.9)	0 (0.0)	0 (0.0)	1 (2.9)	0 (0.0)	13 (37.1)
	GCCs	30	10 (33.3)	2 (6.7)	0 (0.0)	4 (13.3)	3 (10.0)	0 (0.0)	0 (0.0)	4 (13.3)	0 (0.0)	11 (36.7)
Biscuits, sweets, and semi-sweets	GFPs	96	34 (35.4)	39 (40.6)	11 (11.5)	41 (42.7)	4 (4.2)	13 (13.5) **	5 (5.2)	15 (15.6)	48 (50.0)	38 (39.6) *
	GCCs	95	39 (41.1)	43 (45.3)	9 (9.5)	42 (44.2)	1 (1.1)	1 (1.1)	1 (1.1)	9 (9.5)	38 (40.0)	52 (54.7)
Pastries and cakes	GFPs	127	95 (74.8)	35 (27.6) *	8 (6.3)	61 (48.4)	7 (5.5)	28 (22.0) ***	17 (13.4)	17 (13.4)	19 (15.0) ***	107 (84.9) ***
	GCCs	116	88 (75.9)	47 (40.9)	3 (2.6)	67 (57.8)	9 (7.8)	0 (0.0)	12 (10.3)	14 (12.1)	0 (0.0)	0 (0.0)
Churros	GFPs	6	2 (33.3)	1 (16.7)	0 (0.0)	0 (0.0)	1 (16.7)	0 (0.0)	1 (16.7)	0 (0.0)	0 (0.0)	0 (0.0)
	GCCs	6	2 (33.3)	0 (0.0)	0 (0.0)	0 (0.0)	0 (0.0)	0 (0.0)	1 (16.7)	0 (0.0)	0 (0.0)	2 (33.3)

Results are expressed as frequency (*n*) of products, including a specific ingredient, and percentage based on the total products within the group. * $p < 0.05$ ** $p < 0.01$ *** $p < 0.001$ gluten-free products (GFPs) vs. gluten-containing counterparts (GCCs) within the same food group. Cocoa: cocoa oil, cocoa butter, cocoa, cocoa paste, and chocolate powder. Margarine 1: palm, rapeseed, and emulsifier. Margarine 2: coconut and sunflower. Animal fat: animal fat, butter, and milk fat. Emulsifiers: mono- and diglycerides of fatty acids and sunflower, soy, and rapeseed lecithin.

Table 4. Types of sugars and sweeteners and frequency of use in the formulation of gluten-free and gluten-containing products commonly consumed for breakfast.

Breakfast Product		*n*	Sucrose *n* (%)	Dextrose *n* (%)	Glucose and Fructose Syrup *n* (%)	Non-Refined or Cane Sugar *n* (%)	Rice Syrup *n* (%)	Beetroot Sugar Syrup *n* (%)	Honey *n* (%)	Lactose *n* (%)	Other Sugars *n* (%)	Low Calorie Sweetener *n* (%)
Bread and similar	GFPs	100	45 (45.0)	32 (32.0) ***	11 (11.0)	8 (8.0) *	22 (22.0) ***	1 (1.0)	5 (5.0) *	1 (1.0)	51 (51.0) ***	0 (0.0)
	GCCs	101	45 (44.6)	4 (4.0)	4 (4.0)	2 (2.0)	1 (1.0)	0 (0.0)	0 (0.0)	0 (0.0)	10 (9.9)	0 (0.0)
Breakfast cereals	GFPs	35	23 (65.7)	2 (5.7)	4 (11.4) **	6 (17.1)	1 (2.9)	0 (0.0)	1 (2.9) *	1 (2.9)	8 (22.9) ***	1 (2.9)
	GCCs	30	25 (83.3)	1 (3.3)	12 (40.0)	5 (16.7)	0 (0.0)	0 (0.0)	6 (20.0)	0 (0.0)	21 (70.0)	0 (0.0)
Biscuits, sweets, and semi-sweets	GFPs	96	82 (85.4)	15 (15.6)	32 (33.3) ***	20(31.7) ***	1 (1.0)	9 (9.4) **	2 (2.1)	29(30.2) **	46 (59.7)	4 (4.2)
	GCCs	95	81 (85.3)	12 (12.6)	0 (0.0)	6 (6.3)	0 (0.0)	0 (0.0)	2 (2.1)	48 (50.5)	57 (60.0)	6 (6.3)
Pastries and cakes	GFPs	127	114 (89.8)	49 (38.6) **	61 (48.0)	6 (4.7)	3 (2.4)	0 (0.0)	1 (0.8)	6 (4.7) *	95 (74.8) *	15 (11.8) *
	GCCs	116	108 (93.1)	27 (23.3)	63 (54.3)	2 (1.7)	0 (0.0)	0 (0.0)	3 (2.6)	0 (0.0)	73 (62.9)	25 (21.6)
Churros	GFPs	6	0 (0.0)	2 (33.3)	0 (0.0)	0 (0.0)	0 (0.0)	0 (0.0)	0 (0.0)	0 (0.0)	2 (33.3)	0 (0.0)
	GCCs	6	1 (16.7)	2 (33.3)	0 (0.0)	0 (0.0)	0 (0.0)	0 (0.0)	0 (0.0)	0 (0.0)	3 (50.0)	0 (0.0)

Results are expressed as frequency (*n*) of products, including a specific ingredient and percentage based on the total products within the group. * $p < 0.05$ ** $p < 0.01$ *** $p < 0.001$ gluten-free products (GFPs) vs. gluten-containing counterparts (GCCs) within the same food group. Non-refined or cane sugar: molasses, cane sugar, and cane sugar syrup. Lactose: lactose and milk powder. Other sugars: isomaltose, fructose, glucose, agave syrup, corn syrup, barley malt extract, caramelised sugar syrup, invert sugar syrup, and liquid caramel.

Table 5. Types of fibres and frequency of use in the formulation of gluten-free and gluten-containing products commonly consumed for breakfast.

Breakfast Product		n	Hydroxypropyl Methyl Cellulose n (%)	Xanthan Gum n (%)	Guar Gum n (%)	Gum n (%)	Psyllium Bamboo n (%)	Sodium Carboxymethyl Cellulose n (%)	Pectin n (%)	Other Fibres n (%)	Oat Fibre Wheat Bran n (%)
Bread and similar	GFPs	100	67 (67.0) ***	48 (48.0) ***	14 (14.0)	36 (36.0) *	48 (48.0) ***	14 (14.0) **	11 (12.4)	19 (19.8) ***	0 (0.0) ***
	GCCs	101	5 (5.0)	6 (5.9)	17 (16.8)	23 (22.8)	3 (3.0)	3 (3.0)	1 (7.7)	4 (4.0)	13 (12.9)
Breakfast cereals	GFPs	35	0 (0.0)	0 (0.0)	0 (0.0)	0 (0.0)	1 (2.9)	0 (0.0)	0 (0.0)	1 (3.1)	0 (0.0) *
	GCCs	30	0 (0.0)	0 (0.0)	0 (0.0)	0 (0.0)	0 (0.0)	0 (0.0)	0 (0.0)	0 (0.0)	5 (16.7)
Biscuits, sweets, and semi-sweets	GFPs	96	0 (0.0)	23 (24.0) ***	20 (20.8) ***	4 (4.2)	0 (0.0)	0 (0.0)	11 (18.0)	0 (0.0)	0 (0.0)
	GCCs	95	0 (0.0)	0 (0.0)	1 (1.1)	2 (2.1)	0 (0.0)	0 (0.0)	8 (8.4)	0 (0.0)	0 (0.0)
Pastries and cakes	GFPs	127	31 (24.4) ***	91 (71.7) ***	26 (20.5) *	98 (77.2) ***	16 (12.6) ***	13 (10.2) **	9 (7.1) **	4 (4.0) *	0 (0.0)
	GCCs	116	0 (0.0)	22 (19.0)	13 (11.2)	0 (0.0)	0 (0.0)	2 (1.7)	0 (0.0)	0 (0.0)	0 (0.0)
Churros	GFPs	6	0 (0.0)	2 (33.3)	1 (16.7)	0 (0.0)	0 (0.0)	0 (0.0)	0 (0.0)	0 (0.0)	0 (0.0)
	GCCs	6	0 (0.0)	1 (16.7)	0 (0.0)	1 (16.7)	0 (0.0)	0 (0.0)	0 (0.0)	0 (0.0)	0 (0.0)

Results are expressed as frequency (n) of products, including a specific ingredient, and percentage based on the total products within the group. * $p < 0.05$ ** $p < 0.01$ *** $p < 0.001$ gluten-free products (GFPs) vs. gluten-containing counterparts (GCCs) within the same food group. Gum: unspecified gum. Pectin: pectin, fibre of apple, banana, and citrus. Other fibres: chicory, potato, rice, pea, soy fibre and rice, and pea bran.

Table 6. Energy and nutrient composition per 100 g of gluten-free and gluten-containing breakfast products, according to labelling nutritional information.

Breakfast Products		n	Energy (kcal)	Fats (g)	Saturated Fat (g)	Carbohydrates (g)	Sugars (g)	Protein (g)	Fibre (g)	Salt (g)
Bread and similar	GFPs	100	294.9 ± 57.8	5.6 ± 3.4 *	2.2 ± 2.6 *	55.6 ± 14.2	5.1 ± 3.3 *	3.0 ± 1.9 *	5.6 ± 2.1 *	1.4 ± 0.5 *
	GCCs	101	288.4 ± 52.1	4.0 ± 3.4	1.1 ± 1.4	52.8 ± 12.1	3.9 ± 2.9	9.2 ± 2.8	3.9 ± 2.2	1.3 ± 0.4
Breakfast cereals	GFPs	35	385.1 ± 26.5	4.5 ± 4.5	1.3 ± 1.4	75.6 ± 9.3	15.4 ± 10.8	7.9 ± 2.6	5.3 ± 3.4	0.6 ± 0.6
	GCCs	30	388.5 ± 29.9	6.0 ± 5.2	2.0 ± 2.4	71.4 ± 10.1	19.4 ± 9.5	8.7 ± 2.3	6.9 ± 4.7	0.6 ± 0.4
Biscuits, sweets, and semi-sweets	GFPs	96	471.5 ± 41.8	19.9 ± 6.0	9.4 ± 5.5	67.5 ± 6.4 *	25.5 ± 8.4	4.4 ± 1.5 *	3.9 ± 4.8	0.6 ± 0.5
	GCCs	95	469.3 ± 48.7	20.0 ± 5.8	8.7 ± 5.9	65.1 ± 7.4	26.9 ± 10.6	6.3 ± 1.4	3.5 ± 2.0	0.7 ± 0.4
Pastries and cakes	GFPs	127	400.7 ± 71.4 *	21.5 ± 6.9	7.3 ± 5.1	47.0 ± 8.2	20.5 ± 8.8 *	4.1 ± 1.8 *	3.0 ± 1.7 *	0.8 ± 0.6 *
	GCCs	116	427.0 ± 72.9	22.5 ± 6.7	8.7 ± 6.1	52.1 ± 34.9	23.7 ± 10.6	5.6 ±1.5	2.3 ± 1.4	0.6 ± 0.3
Churros	GFPs	6	237.9 ± 122.2	9.3 ± 8.7	3.5 ± 4.2	36.6 ± 11.1	6.5 ± 10.9	1.7 ± 1.6 *	-	0.8 ± 0.2 *
	GCCs	6	201.5 ± 115.6	4.1 ± 8.3	1.8 ± 4.0	35.0 ± 10.4	8.6 ± 10.3	5.2 ± 0.9	2.0 ± 0.3	17.3 ± 39.5

Data are expressed as average ± standard deviation. * $p < 0.05$ gluten-free products (GFPs) vs. gluten-containing counterparts (GCCs) within the same food group.

3.3. Food Habits and Nutrient Intakes for Breakfast

Table 7 shows the daily intake of energy, macronutrients, fibre and salt in Spanish children and adolescents with CD compared to controls, obtained from both the total diet and from breakfast only. The percentage contribution of the energy and nutrient intake for breakfast to total daily intake is also provided. Children and adolescents with CD consumed significantly less energy at breakfast as compared to controls, and the contribution of breakfast to the total daily energy was also slightly lower (19 vs. 20%), although not significantly. Similarly, the intake of saturated fatty acids in breakfast and the contribution of this meal to total saturated fatty acid intakes was smaller in CD. On the other hand, breakfast had a higher contribution to total salt intake in the infant–juvenile celiac population, but daily salt intake was significantly lower compared to controls. As for protein, daily intake and protein contained in breakfast were lower in children and adolescents with CD. We found no differences in carbohydrates, sugars, or fibre intakes.

Table 7. Contribution of gluten-free and gluten-containing breakfast products to the diet (energy and nutrient content) and macronutrient distribution for total daily energy intake and energy from breakfast in Spanish children and adolescents with celiac disease.

	Total Daily Intake		**Intake from Breakfast**		**% Contribution of Breakfast**	
	CD $n = 70$	**CONTROL** $n = 67$	**CD** $n = 70$	**CONTROL** $n = 67$	**CD** $n = 70$	**CONTROL** $n = 67$
Energy (kcal/day)	2043.0 ± 449.1	2121.4 ± 469.4	370.0 ± 107.2 *	411.7 ± 115.8	18.8 ± 6.5	20.1 ± 6.7
Fats (g/day)	93.9 ± 20.1	99.1 ± 26.8	14.0 ± 6.3 *	16.2 ± 7.0	15.5 ± 7.6	17.4 ± 8.6
% Energy from fats	41.9 ± 6.4	42.4 ± 7.8	34.1 ± 9.0	34.5 ± 9.0		
Saturated fat (g/day)	32.0 ± 7.9	33.8 ± 10.0	6.3 ± 3.1 *	7.8 ± 3.5	20.2 ± 9.7 *	24.9 ± 12.4
% Energy from saturated fat	14.3 ± 2.5	14.1 ± 3.3	15.1 ± 5.4	16.7 ± 5.3		
Carbohydrates (g/day)	208.8 ± 66.6	216.5 ± 57.6	49.5 ± 15.3	52.1 ± 15.2	25.4 ± 10.0	24.9 ± 7.5
% Energy from carbohydrates	40.6 ± 7.0	40.9 ± 6.6	53.9 ± 7.7 *	51.1 ± 7.3		
Sugars (g/day)	88.5 ± 25.3	88.5 ± 26.6	27.1 ± 10.5	30.4 ± 11.2	32.2 ± 13.5	35.9 ± 13.5
Protein (g/day)	77.4 ± 18.1 *	89.0 ± 20.5	10.30 ± 2.6 *	13.0 ± 4.0	14.1 ± 5.2	15.1 ± 5.0
% Energy from protein	15.2 ± 2.2 *	16.8 ± 2.5	11.6 ± 3.7 *	13.1 ± 3.0		
Fibre (g/day)	18.0 ± 7.6	16.9 ± 5.5	2.6 ± 1.5	2.5 ± 1.1	15.9 ± 9.3	15.6 ± 8.1
Salt (g/day)	4.5 ± 2.4 *	5.4 ± 2.2	0.9 ± 0.4	0.8 ± 0.5	23.5 ± 12.6 *	16.2 ± 8.2

Data are expressed as average ± standard deviation. * $p < 0.05$ children and adolescents with celiac disease (CD) vs. control.

Table 7 also represents the macronutrient distribution for total daily energy intake and for the energy obtained from breakfast in children and adolescents with CD. Macronutrient contribution to total daily energy intake in both groups was similar, except for protein, which was lower in the case of participants with CD. In the case of breakfast, carbohydrates provided a higher proportion of energy and a lower amount of proteins in participants with CD, as compared to controls.

Table 8 shows the type of products consumed for breakfast by Spanish children and adolescents with CD compared to controls. The four main food groups most frequently consumed at breakfast were grain products, sugars, sweets and pastries, milk and dairy products, and fruits, and there were no significant differences between CD and controls. However, the consumption of eggs and derivatives was more frequent among children and adolescents with CD.

Table 9 shows the contribution of the four main breakfast food groups (grain products, fruits, dairies, sugars, sweets, and confectionery) to the energy and nutrients provided by this meal in both children and adolescents with CD and controls. The other food groups consumed at breakfast (eggs, meat products, vegetables, oils, etc.) contribute only a small proportion of the energy and nutrients and are, therefore, not shown. The percentage of energy and nutrients provided by fruits at breakfast was very similar between participants with CD and controls. Milk and dairy products contributed more to saturated fat and protein intakes at breakfast, and less to the salt intake in the CD group as compared to controls. Major differences were found in the grain products (grains and flours, breakfast cereals, breads, biscuits, and baked goods) and sugars, sweets, and confectionery (sugars, jams, chocolates, sweets, and pastries). The products belonging to the group of sugars, sweets, and confectionery contribute to energy and nutrient intakes in breakfast at a greater extent for the group of children and adolescents with CD and, in contrast, foods from the grain products group contribute more extensively for the control group. Therefore, although the total amount of carbohydrates and simple sugars consumed at breakfast was similar between the two groups, their origin and nature are different.

Table 8. Food groups consumed for breakfast by Spanish children and adolescents with celiac disease.

Food Groups	CD $n = 70$	CONTROL $n = 67$
Grains (n (%))	67 (95.7)	67 (100.0)
Sugars, sweets, and pastries (n (%))	59 (84.2)	48 (71.6)
Milk and dairy products (n (%))	69 (98.6)	67 (100.0)
Fruits (n (%))	34 (48.6)	35 (52.2)
Legumes (n (%))	2 (2.9)	2 (3.0)
Vegetables (n (%))	6 (8.6)	4 (6.0)
Meat and meat products (n (%))	7 (10.0)	14 (20.9)
Fish and derivatives (n (%))	1 (1.4)	1 (1.5)
Eggs and derivatives (n (%))	7 (10.0)	1 (1.5) *
Oils and fats (n (%))	36 (51.4)	28 (41.8)
Beverages (n (%))	10 (14.0)	4 (6.0)
Readily prepared and precooked meals (n (%))	0	1 (1.5)
Sauces and condiments (n (%))	4 (5.7)	0 *

Results are expressed as frequency (n) number of subjects taking the product and percentage based on the total number of participants. * $p < 0.05$ children and adolescents with celiac disease (CD) vs. control.

Table 9. Contribution of the different food groups to the energy and nutrient content of breakfast in Spanish children and adolescents with celiac disease.

	Intake in Breakfast		% Contribution from Grain Products		% Contribution from Fruits		% Contribution from Dairy		% Contribution from Sugars, Sweets, and Confectionery	
	CD $n = 70$	CONTROL $n = 67$	CD $n = 70$	CONTROL $n = 67$	CD $n = 70$	CONTROL $n = 67$	CD $n = 70$	CONTROL $n = 67$	CD $n = 70$	CONTROL $n = 67$
Energy (kcal/day)	370.0 ± 107.2 *	411.7 ± 115.8	37.0 ± 16.6 *	44.7 ± 17.8	6.4 ± 8.2	6.9 ± 8.7	32.5 ± 13.5	30.6 ± 11.0	16.6 ± 15.6 **	8.7 ± 11.9
Fats (g/day)	14.0 ± 6.3	16.2 ± 7.0	27.3 ± 23.7 *	38.0 ± 25.2	0.9 ± 1.8	1.3 ± 3.9	41.9 ± 25.7	35.1 ± 19.3	13.2 ± 17.7 *	6.2 ± 14.4
Saturated fat (g/day)	6.3 ± 3.1 *	7.8 ± 3.5	19.3 ± 20.1 ***	34.0 ± 23.6	0.2 ± 0.5	0.3 ± 0.8	54.4 ± 27.2 *	44.8 ± 21.7	11.5 ± 15.0 **	5.5 ± 11.4
Carbohydrates (g/day)	49.5 ± 15.3	52.1 ± 15.2	46.3 ± 19.2 *	54.3 ± 18.7	9.9 ± 12.6	11.1 ± 13.7	21.0 ± 9.5	21.6 ± 8.9	21.3 ± 17.8 **	11.8 ± 13.8
Sugars (g/day)	27.1 ± 10.5	30.4 ± 11.2	17.5 ± 12.0 ***	25.5 ± 17.6	16.9 ± 21.1	17.7 ± 21.2	39.5 ± 18.2	38.7 ± 16.7	23.7 ± 18.4 **	16.2 ± 15.5
Protein (g/day)	10.30 ± 2.6 *	13.0 ± 4.0	18.0 ± 10.4 ***	28.1 ± 10.6	3.1± 4.2	3.0 ± 4.4	66.1 ± 15.2 ***	58.8 ± 14.9	7.2 ± 7.6 *	4.4 ± 8.0
Fibre (g/day)	2.6 ± 1.5	2.5 ± 1.1	62.5 ± 27.4 *	74.2 ± 24.7	13.6 ± 18.9	16.6 ± 22.6	0.0 ± 0.0	0.0 ± 0.0	20.7 ± 23.7 ***	8.8 ± 10.4
Salt (g/day)	0.9 ± 0.4	0.8 ± 0.5	41.6 ± 20.9	45.4 ± 16.1	0.3 ± 0.7	0.3 ± 0.4	29.9 ± 14.5 ***	39.9 ± 14.8	18.5 ± 18.5 ***	8.3 ± 8.7

Data are expressed as average ± standard deviation. * $p < 0.05$ ** $p < 0.01$ *** $p < 0.001$ children and adolescents with celiac disease (CD) vs. control.

4. Discussion

In this study, we have extensively analysed the breakfast diet among Spanish children and adolescents with celiac disease (CD) in comparison with a control sample (non-celiac). Most of the children and adolescents evaluated in both groups ate breakfast every day (98.5%). This was a positive observation, since breakfast consumption compared to skipping breakfast has been associated with better nutrient intake in different studies [1,4,7,38–41]. The group of children and adolescents with CD ingested slightly less energy (not significant, 19 vs. 20% of daily energy) than controls. The intake of energy for breakfast in our study is slightly higher, and therefore better, than that reported by Ruiz et al. (2018) in the ANIBES Study on the general Spanish population [2], in which children and teenagers only consumed 18% of daily energy in this meal, and similarly to the data reported by Cuadrado Soto et al. (2020) from the ENALIA Study [1], in which more than half of the children who ate breakfast (56.4%) obtained less than 20% of their daily calories at breakfast, with a mean of 18.3%. According to current Spanish dietary guidelines and the International Breakfast Research Initiative (IBRI) recommendations [18,42], breakfast should provide 15–25% of total energy in the diet (circa 300–500 kcal). Therefore, caloric recommendations for breakfast seem to be accomplished in the assessed population groups in the present study.

In terms of adequacy, the macronutrient distribution for breakfast in CD was balanced (54% of total energy from carbohydrates; 12% from proteins; 34% from lipids), with a higher proportion of energy resulting from carbohydrates and a lower proportion from lipids than that which was obtained for the daily value, and for the control group, but very close to the IBRI recommendations [42]. Therefore, children and adolescents with CD do manage to have a balanced breakfast.

In terms of food variety, various studies indicate that breakfast should include foods from at least three key food groups, namely: starchy foods (cereals, pasta, bread), fruit and vegetables, and milk and dairy products [1,2,42]. In this sense, studies carried out on Spanish children found that breakfast at these ages should be improved. For example, the ALADINO Study [12] showed that breakfasts that included foods from the three recommended groups are scarce (only 2.2% of schoolchildren). In the ENALIA Study [1,2,42], the frequency of consumption of the three types of food is higher (8.4%) but is still insufficient. The present study shows more positive data, since almost half of the population sample of both groups took food from all three basic groups, and 49% of participants with CD and 52% of the control group consumed fruit for breakfast. However, the contribution of fruit to breakfast energy and nutrients is still lower than recommended and is similar between subjects with CD and controls. Milk and its derivatives and cereals were present in 96–100% of breakfasts.

When compared to controls, children and adolescents with CD consume a significantly lower amount of protein, both daily and for breakfast, although it is still enough to cover protein needs. This could be due to the statistically lower protein content of the gluten-free products (GFPs), which is the result of the use of corn and rice flours, and corn starch, which have a low protein and high carbohydrate concentration than wheat flour. These results agree with similar studies that indicated that GFPs, compared to gluten-containing counterparts (GCCs), contain lower protein and higher carbohydrate contents [20,34,43–52]. Breakfast protein is mainly provided by dairy products, especially in celiacs who consume less from cereals, in which gluten is removed. In this sense, some commercialised GFPs have different protein concentrates or isolates (obtained from microorganisms, animals, and plants) that are added to improve both the quality and the nutritional profile of GFPs [53]. It should be noted that, mainly in gluten-free breads, the functionality of the proteins is more relevant than the nutritional properties since trying to mimic the attributes of gluten from diverse protein origins is a technological challenge and a wide research field [52,54–59]. In our study, the CD group also ate significantly more eggs and egg products, which are good sources of protein at breakfast. The addition of eggs at breakfast can contribute to nutrient intakes and overall dietary adequacy and play a role in public health initiatives aimed at increasing the intake of under-consumed nutrients and nutrients of concern [60]. This recommendation could be especially interesting to youngsters with CD since eggs would be very useful in forming the structural doughs through improving the cohesion and elasticity of gluten-free breads when low doses are incorporated, as well as increasing the nutritional value [54,61]. Eggs are also widely used in gluten-free bakery and confectionery products to technologically compensate for the withdrawal of gluten, and occasionally in gluten-free breads. Similarly, dairy protein sources, such as yoghurt and cheese, are also added as confirmed by results from other studies [57,61]. In addition, an adequate protein intake could be an advantage in terms of inducing greater satiety and avoiding possible snacking with unsuitable foods in the mid-morning meal.

GFPs may have a lower protein content, but thanks to them, children and adolescents with CD manage to consume enough carbohydrates and fibre in their breakfast, with even a significantly higher contribution of carbohydrates as compared to controls, although they do have to avoid common cereal-based products. The mean carbohydrate and sugar contents of breakfast GFPs were like those of GCCs, except for slightly higher amounts of total carbohydrate in gluten-free biscuits, sweets and semi-sweets and sugars in bread and similar [44,50,52]. Only a few studies have revealed a lower content in total carbohydrates and sugars with significant differences of gluten-free cakes, muffins, pastries, and biscuits compared to those made with wheat flour [62]. As for fibre, it is a common and widespread ingredient used in the formulation of GFPs [52,54,63], as we have demonstrated in this study. Incorporating foreign fibres, or ingredients with a high fibre content, has significantly improved the nutritional composition of GFPs since the offer of commercial gluten-free whole-grain products is very unusual [56]. Pseudo-cereals such as amaranth, buckwheat, and quinoa, but also milled legumes, seeds, and nuts, are optional ingredients increasingly used for the preparation of gluten-free baked goods compared to GCCs [54,56,64], which enlarge the quantity of fibre of the GFPs. Nevertheless, despite the higher fibre content of GFPs, people following a strict GFD have a lower fibre intake than the rest of the population if the intake of the whole day, not only for breakfast, is assessed [27,36,45,65].

Moreover, the intake of saturated fatty acids (SFA) at breakfast appears to be lower in the celiac group, although there is no difference in the intake of these fatty acids in the total diet compared to the non-celiac group, indicating a possible "intake compensation" with other meals of the day. Furthermore, the contribution of SFA to total daily energy intake and that provided for breakfast is similar between the two groups. In this respect, it is important to point out that the content of SFA in cereal-based GFPs depends on the type of oil/fat used for its preparation [43]. In our study of ingredients, we found that the use of polyunsaturated fats, such as sunflower or olive oils, is frequent in breads and pastries and cakes, but the use of saturated fat, such as palm and cocoa is also frequent in pastries and cakes and biscuits, sweets, and semi-sweets. Results are in accordance with most of the previous studies [44,46,47,52,66]. Therefore, saturated fat intake in breakfast in CD may highly depend on the type of products chosen. In addition, it should be noted that the foods that contribute most to the intake of SFA in the celiac group are milk and dairy derivatives, and this food group appears to have a beneficial effect on cardiometabolic risk factors, compared to other sources of SFA [67].

There are some areas for improvement in the formulation of gluten-free breakfast products and in the general habits and food choices for breakfast in children and adolescents with CD [44,45,54,68]. For example, the consumption of carbohydrates, sugars, and fibre was similar in both types of breakfast and is mainly provided by cereals, but celiacs obtained a higher proportion of the aforementioned nutrients from the group of sugars, sweets, and confectionary, and less from grain products, which changes the type of ingredients/nutrients they consume. Generally, the gluten-free diet is rich in products with a high glycaemic index (GI), which increases the development of chronic diseases. In this context, it is also important that these products have high amounts of protein and fibre to lower the GI. It is recommended that the addition of whole grain flours, or pseudocereals and legume could enhance the nutritional quality of GFPs [69]. The products marketed as GFPs, evaluated in our study, were more frequently added with sugars such as dextrose, the syrup of glucose, and non-refined or cane sugar, rice syrup, etc. The inclusion of these sugars, as a fermentable ingredient in GFPs, compensate for the lack of hydrolytic enzymes in starch-based preparations [52]. In contrast, in GCPs, sugars often result from the activity of amylase enzymes on starch. In addition, sugar in GFPs enhances the aroma due to non-enzymatic browning reactions [70]. It is known that, in GCPs, sugar, and also fat, hinder the gluten network [52]. If a diet should require avoiding grain-based products because of their gluten content, children and adolescents could make healthier choices of carbohydrates and fibre sources that provide less sugars, such as nuts, dried fruit, date, or peanut pastes. Added sugars are key nutrients in product reformulation which should be focussed on [52].

According to the total diet data, celiac children and adolescents consume significantly less salt than controls; however, at breakfast, the salt intake is higher. An analysis of products marketed as gluten-free indicates that most of them have a higher salt content, especially breads, pastries, and cakes, compared to GCCs [44,71,72]. Salt reduction in cereal-based products for celiacs is another important issue to be addressed by the food industry, as we have previously proposed [27].

In our view, the nutritional quality of the gluten-free breakfast could also improve with nutrition education, especially focusing children and teenagers with CD. Actual consumption trends in CD warrant the need to promote the consumption of unprocessed GFPs such as pseudocereals, with better nutritional quality, and homemade products with flours different to rice or corn, together with proper nutritional guidance, including the avoidance of manufactured GFPs. The challenge in using unconventional flours in food preparations is the need for high food literacy (e.g., food skills, budgeting, and nutrition knowledge) and more time for meal planning and cooking in comparison to purchasing ready-to-eat products. It would also be helpful to include foods of a different nature, such as more fruits, other sources of protein, and products derived from legumes and nuts.

Strengths and Limitations

It is the first time that such a detailed study of breakfast in children and adolescents with CD has been carried out, both in terms of food, ingredients, and nutrients. Only by conducting this analysis can differences in the type and nature of nutrients be observed, which could be used to assess the quality of breakfasts and to establish new indices in the future.

Unfortunately, we have not been able to analyse the micronutrient intake of breakfast in both groups, celiacs and controls, since micronutrient content is not specified on the labelling of GFPs. Because GFPs constitute an important part of the diet of young people with CD (they provide up to a quarter of the daily energy), we would be significantly underestimating the micronutrient intake. Another limitation of the study was the small sample size, because the research is a follow-up analysis of an initial study comparing the dietary habits of children diagnosed with CD, and the sample size was adapted to the present study to compare breakfast habits and nutritional quality. Future studies which include a larger sample size will further contribute to this area of research.

5. Conclusions

The present study provides information on the type of breakfast eaten by a sample of Spanish children and adolescents with celiac disease (CD) compared to children of the same age without the disease (controls). Until now, breakfast has not been evaluated in this population group and, according to the literature, this meal is related to a better nutritional status, the prevention of cardiometabolic diseases, and the improvement of cognitive performance. Relevant positive issues were observed, such as that virtually no one skips breakfast, and almost half of the sample includes all three recommended food groups (cereals, dairy, and fruits). The energy intake and the distribution of macronutrients is quite adequate. However, there are also many areas for improvement. For example, the cereal-based gluten-free products that are normally included in breakfasts in our study are almost 100% manufactured by the food industry. Thus, we observed that although commercial gluten-free products (GFPs) contribute to an adequate intake of carbohydrates and fibre, they also provide less protein and more added sugars than GCCs. Moreover, the group with CD has a higher intake of nutrients from the group of "sugars, sweets, and confectionary" than those provided by grain products. To compensate for the low protein intake from this source, celiacs consume more protein from dairy products and seem to include more eggs in this meal of the day compared to controls.

Author Contributions: Conceptualization, E.A.-A. and N.Ú.; data curation, M.P.G.; formal analysis, M.P.G. and N.Ú.; funding acquisition, E.A.-A.; investigation, C.B.-F., V.F., M.A. and Á.G.-G.; methodology, M.P.G.; project administration, E.A.-A.; resources, E.A.-A. and N.Ú.; supervision, E.A.-A.; validation, M.P.G., E.A.-A. and N.Ú.; writing—original draft, N.Ú., M.P.G., V.F.; writing—review and editing, E.A.-A. All authors have read and agreed to the published version of the manuscript.

Funding: This research was funded by Universidad San Pablo-CEU, CEU Universities: II call grants for recognized research groups. Grant code MGI21EAA.

Institutional Review Board Statement: The study was conducted in accordance with the Declaration of Helsinki n Ethical Principles for Medical Research involving Human Subjects (revised in October 2008) and approved by the Ethics Committee for Human Studies of Universidad San Pablo-CEU (Authorization number 102–15).

Informed Consent Statement: Informed consent was obtained from all subjects and guardians, or caregivers involved in the study.

Data Availability Statement: The data on gluten-free food composition used in this study are openly available in the institutional repository at Universidad San Pablo-CEU (CEU Repositorio Institucional) at http://hdl.handle.net/10637/13562 (Last accessed on 15 November 2022). The data on dietary intakes presented in this study are available upon request from the corresponding author.

Acknowledgments: We acknowledge the Celiac Disease Patient Association in Madrid, Spain (Asociación de Celíacos y Sensibles al Gluten de Madrid), for their contribution in spreading the recruitment call.

Conflicts of Interest: The authors declare no conflict of interest. The funders had no role in the design of the study; in the collection, analyses, or interpretation of data; in the writing of the manuscript; or in the decision to publish the results.

Abbreviations

ANIBES: Anthropometry, Intake and Energy Balance Study; ALADINO: Food, Physical Activity, Child development and Obesity Study; CD: celiac disease; ENALIA: National Dietary Survey on the Child and Adolescent Population Study; GCCs: gluten-containing counterparts; GFD: gluten-free diet; GFPs: gluten-free products; HELENA: Healthy Lifestyle in Europe by Nutrition in Adolescence Study; HOMA-IR: homeostasis model assessment—insulin resistance; IBRI: International Breakfast Research Initiative; OW/OB: Overweight/obesity; SFA: Saturated fatty acids; SENC: Spanish Society of Community Nutrition (Sociedad Española de Nutrición Comunitaria).

References

1. Cuadrado-Soto, E.; López-Sobaler, A.M.; Jiménez-Ortega, A.I.; Bermejo, L.M.; Aparicio, A.; Ortega, R.M. Breakfast habits of a representative sample of the Spanish child and adolescent population (The ENALIA Study): Association with diet quality. *Nutrients* **2020**, *12*, 3772. [CrossRef] [PubMed]
2. Ruiz, E.; Ávila, J.M.; Valero, T.; Rodriguez, P.; Varela-Moreiras, G. Breakfast consumption in Spain: Patterns, nutrient intake and quality. Findings from the ANIBES Study, a study from the International Breakfast Research Initiative. *Nutrients* **2018**, *10*, 1324. [CrossRef] [PubMed]
3. Alexy, U.; Wicher, M.; Kersting, M. Breakfast trends in children and adolescents: Frequency and quality. *Public Health Nutr.* **2010**, *13*, 1795–1802. [CrossRef] [PubMed]

4. Moreno-Aznar, L.A.; Vidal Carou, M.D.C.; López Sobaler, A.M.; Varela-Moreiras, G.; Moreno Villares, J.M. Role of breakfast and its quality in the health of children and adolescents in Spain. *Nutr. Hosp.* **2021**, *38*, 396–409. [CrossRef] [PubMed]
5. Grupo Colaborativo de la Sociedad Española de Nutrición Comunitaria (SENC); Bartrina, J.A.; Val, V.A.; Aldalur, E.M.; Muñoz, E.M.d.C.; Anta, R.M.O.; Pérez-Rodrigo, C.; Izquierdo, J.Q.; Martín, A.R.; Viñas, B.R.; et al. Guías alimentarias para la población española (SENC, diciembre 2016): La nueva pirámide de la alimentación saludable. *Nutr. Hosp.* **2016**, *33*, 1–48.
6. Sincovich, A.; Moller, H.; Smithers, L.; Brushe, M.; Lassi, Z.S.; Brinkman, S.A.; Gregory, T. Prevalence of breakfast skipping among children and adolescents: A cross-sectional population level study. *BMC Pediatr.* **2022**, *22*, 220. [CrossRef]
7. Ardeshirlarijani, E.; Namazi, N.; Jabbari, M.; Zeinali, M.; Gerami, H.; Jalili, R.Z.; Larijani, B.; Azadbakht, L. The link between breakfast skipping and overweigh/obesity in children and adolescents: A meta-analysis of observational studies. *J. Diabetes Metab. Disord.* **2019**, *18*, 657–664. [CrossRef]
8. Szajewska, H.; Ruszczynski, M. Systematic review demonstrating that breakfast consumption influences body weight outcomes in children and adolescents in Europe. *Crit. Rev. Food Sci. Nutr.* **2010**, *50*, 113–119. [CrossRef]
9. Rani, R.; Dharaiya, C.N.; Singh, B. Importance of not skipping breakfast: A review. *Int. J. Food Sci. Technol.* **2021**, *56*, 28–38. [CrossRef]
10. Souza, M.R.; Neves, M.E.A.; Gorgulho, B.M.; Souza, A.M.; Nogueira, P.S.; Ferreira, M.G.; Rodrigues, P.R.M. Breakfast skipping and cardiometabolic risk factors in adolescents: Systematic review. *Rev. Saude Publica* **2021**, *55*, 107. [CrossRef]
11. Hallström, L.; Labayen, I.; Ruiz, J.R.; Patterson, E.; Vereecken, C.A.; Breidenassel, C.; Gottrand, F.; Huybrechts, I.; Manios, Y.; Mistura, L.; et al. Breakfast consumption and CVD risk factors in European adolescents: The HELENA (Healthy Lifestyle in Europe by Nutrition in Adolescence) Study. *Public Health Nutr.* **2013**, *16*, 1296–1305. [CrossRef]
12. Agencia, Española de Consumo, Seguridad Alimentaria y Nutrición; Ministerio de Sanidad, Servicios Sociales e Igualdad. Estudio de Vigilancia del Crecimiento, Alimentación, Actividad Física, Desarrollo Infantil y Obesidad en España 2015. Madrid, España, 2016. Available online: http://www.aecosan.msssi.gob.es/AECOSAN/docs/documentos/nutricion/observatorio/Estudio_ALADINO_2015.pdf (accessed on 10 August 2022).
13. Giménez-Legarre, N.; Santaliestra-Pasías, A.M.; De Henauw, S.; Forsner, M.; González-Gross, M.; Jurado-Fasoli, L.; Kafatos, A.; Karaglani, E.; Lambrinou, C.P.; Molnár, D.; et al. Breakfast consumption and its relationship with diet quality and adherence to Mediterranean diet in European adolescents: The HELENA study. *Eur. J. Clin. Nutr.* **2022**, *76*, 1690–1696. [CrossRef] [PubMed]
14. Lukomskyj, N.; Shi, Y.; Allman-Farinelli, M.; Rangan, A. Associations between breakfast consumption from childhood to adulthood and cardiometabolic health: A systematic review. *Nutr. Diet.* **2021**, *78*, 6–23. [CrossRef]
15. Salas-González, M.D.; Lozano-Estevan, M.D.C.; Aparicio, A.; Bermejo, L.M.; Loria-Kohen, V.; Ortega, R.M.; López-Sobaler, A.M. Breakfast quality and insulin resistance in Spanish schoolchildren: A Cross-Sectional Study. *Int. J. Environ. Res. Public Health* **2023**, *20*, 1181. [CrossRef] [PubMed]
16. Moller, H.; Sincovich, A.; Gregory, T.; Smithers, L. Breakfast skipping and cognitive and emotional engagement at school: A cross-sectional population-level study. *Public Health Nutr.* **2021**, *25*, 3356–3365. [CrossRef]
17. Burrows, T.L.; Whatnall, M.C.; Patterson, A.J.; Hutchesson, M.J. Associations between dietary intake and academic achievement in college students: A systematic review. *Healthcare* **2017**, *5*, 60. [CrossRef] [PubMed]
18. Gibney, M.J.; Barr, S.I.; Bellisle, F.; Drewnowski, A.; Fagt, S.; Livingstone, B.; Masset, G.; Varela Moreiras, G.; Moreno, L.A.; Smith, J.; et al. Breakfast in human nutrition: The International Breakfast Research Initiative. *Nutrients* **2018**, *10*, 559. [CrossRef] [PubMed]
19. López-Sobaler, A.; Cuadrado-Soto, E.; Peral-Suárez, Á.; Aparicio, A.; Ortega, R. Importance of breakfast in the nutritional and health improvement of the population. *Nutr. Hosp.* **2018**, *35*, 3–6. [CrossRef]
20. Mármol-Soler, C.; Matias, S.; Miranda, J.; Larretxi, I.; Fernández-Gil, M.D.P.; Bustamante, M.; Churruca, I.; Martínez, O.; Simón, E. Gluten-free products: Do we need to update our knowledge? *Foods* **2022**, *11*, 3839. [CrossRef]
21. Makharia, G.K.; Chauhan, A.; Singh, P.; Ahuja, V. Review article: Epidemiology of coeliac disease. *Aliment. Pharmacol. Ther.* **2022**, *56*, s3–s17. [CrossRef] [PubMed]
22. King, J.A.; Jeong, J.; Underwood, F.E.; Quan, J.; Panaccione, N.; Windsor, J.W.; Coward, S.; deBruyn, J.; Ronksley, P.E.; Shaheen, A.-A.; et al. Incidence of celiac disease is increasing over time: A systematic review and meta-analysis. *Am. J. Gastroenterol.* **2020**, *115*, 507–525. [CrossRef] [PubMed]
23. Mariné, M.; Farre, C.; Alsina, M.; Vilar, P.; Cortijo, M.; Salas, A.; Fernández-Bañares, F.; Rosinach, M.; Santaolalla, R.; Loras, C.; et al. The prevalence of coeliac disease is significantly higher in children compared with adults. *Aliment. Pharmacol. Ther.* **2011**, *33*, 477–486. [CrossRef]
24. Cilleruelo, M.L.; Roman-Riechmann, E.; Sanchez-Valverde, F.; Donat, E.; Manuel-Ramos, J.; Martín-Orte, E.; López, M.J.; García-Novo, D.; García, S.; Pavón, P.; et al. Spanish national registry of celiac disease: Incidence and clinical presentation. *J. Pediatr. Gastroenterol. Nutr.* **2014**, *59*, 522–526. [CrossRef] [PubMed]
25. Singh, P.; Arora, A.; Strand, T.A.; Leffler, D.A.; Catassi, C.; Green, P.H.; Kelly, C.P.; Ahuja, V.; Makharia, G.K. Global prevalence of celiac disease: Systematic review and meta-analysis. *Clin. Gastroenterol. Hepatol.* **2018**, *16*, 823–836.e822. [CrossRef] [PubMed]
26. Sahin, Y. Celiac disease in children: A review of the literature. *World J. Clin. Pediatr.* **2021**, *10*, 53–71. [CrossRef]
27. González, M.P.; Ballestero-Fernández, C.; Fajardo, V.; Achón, M.; García-González, Á.; Alonso-Aperte, E.; Úbeda, N. Gluten-free product contribution to energy and macronutrient intakes in Spanish children and adolescents with celiac disease. *Foods* **2022**, *11*, 3790. [CrossRef]

28. Akobeng, A.K.; Singh, P.; Kumar, M.; Al Khodor, S. Role of the gut microbiota in the pathogenesis of coeliac disease and potential therapeutic implications. *Eur. J. Nutr.* **2020**, *59*, 3369–3390. [CrossRef]
29. Anania, C.; Pacifico, L.; Olivero, F.; Perla, F.M.; Chiesa, C. Cardiometabolic risk factors in children with celiac disease on a gluten-free diet. *World J. Clin. Pediatr.* **2017**, *6*, 143–148. [CrossRef]
30. Capriati, T.; Francavilla, R.; Ferretti, F.; Castellaneta, S.; Ancinelli, M.; Diamanti, A. The overweight: A rare presentation of celiac disease. *Eur. J. Clin. Nutr.* **2016**, *70*, 282–284. [CrossRef]
31. Assa, A.; Frenkel-Nir, Y.; Tzur, D.; Katz, L.H.; Shamir, R. Cardiovascular risk factors in adolescents with celiac disease: A cross-sectional population-based study. *J. Pediatr. Gastroenterol. Nutr.* **2017**, *65*, 190–194. [CrossRef]
32. Albuquerque, T.G.; Bragotto, A.P.A.; Costa, H.S. Processed food: Nutrition, safety, and public health. *Int. J. Environ. Res. Public Health* **2022**, *19*, 16410. [CrossRef] [PubMed]
33. Fajardo, V.; González, M.P.; Martínez, M.; Samaniego-Vaesken, M.d.L.; Achón, M.; Úbeda, N.; Alonso-Aperte, E. Gluten-Free Food Composition Database (GLUTENFREE-2019). CEU Rel (Institutional Repository). Available online: http://hdl.handle.net/10637/13562 (accessed on 15 November 2022).
34. Fajardo, V.; González, M.P.; Martínez, M.; Samaniego-Vaesken, M.d.L.; Achón, M.; Úbeda, N.; Alonso-Aperte, E. Updated Food composition database for cereal-based gluten free products in Spain: Is reformulation moving on? *Nutrients* **2020**, *12*, 2369. [CrossRef] [PubMed]
35. Authority, E.F.S. Guidance on the EU Menu methodology. *EFSA J.* **2014**, *12*, 3944. [CrossRef]
36. Ballestero, C.; Varela-Moreiras, G.; Úbeda, N.; Alonso-Aperte, E. Nutritional status in Spanish children and adolescents with celiac disease on a gluten free diet compared to non-celiac disease controls. *Nutrients* **2019**, *11*, 2329. [CrossRef]
37. Ortega, R.; López-Sobaler, A.M.; Andrés, P.; Requejo, A.M.; Aparicio, A.; Molinero, L.M. DIAL Program for Dietary Assessment and Food Calculations. Version 3.4.0.9. Dpto. de Nutrición (UCM) y Alce Ingeniería, S.L. Madrid, España, 2017. Available online: https://www.alceingenieria.net/nutricion/descarga.htm (accessed on 30 November 2022).
38. Pereira, G.; Carliana, M.; Aparecida, C. Eveningness is associated with skipping breakfast and poor nutritional intake in Brazilian undergraduate students. *Chronobiol. Int.* **2018**, *35*, 358–367. [CrossRef]
39. O'Neil, C.E.; Byrd-Bredbenner, C.; Hayes, D.; Jana, L.; Klinger, S.E.; Stephenson-Martin, S. The role of breakfast in health: Definition and criteria for a quality breakfast. *J. Acad. Nutr. Diet.* **2014**, *114*, S8–S26. [CrossRef]
40. Ramsay, S.A.; Bloch, T.D.; Marriage, B.; Shriver, L.H.; Spees, C.K.; Taylor, C.A. Skipping breakfast is associated with lower diet quality in young US children. *Eur. J. Clin. Nutr.* **2018**, *72*, 548–556. [CrossRef]
41. Afeiche, M.C.; Taillie, L.S.; Hopkins, S.; Eldridge, A.L.; Popkin, B.M. Breakfast dietary patterns among Mexican children are related to total-day diet quality. *J. Nutr.* **2017**, *147*, 404–412. [CrossRef]
42. Gibney, M.J.; Barr, S.I.; Bellisle, F.; Drewnowski, A.; Fagt, S.; Hopkins, S.; Livingstone, B.; Varela-Moreiras, G.; Moreno, L.; Smith, J.; et al. Towards an evidence-based recommendation for a balanced breakfast—A proposal from the International Breakfast Research Initiative. *Nutrients* **2018**, *10*, 1540. [CrossRef]
43. Calvo-Lerma, J.; Crespo-Escobar, P.; Martinez-Barona, S.; Fornes-Ferrer, V.; Donat, E.; Ribes-Koninckx, C. Differences in the macronutrient and dietary fibre profile of gluten-free products as compared to their gluten-containing counterparts. *Eur. J. Clin. Nutr.* **2019**, *73*, 930–936. [CrossRef]
44. Miranda, J.; Lasa, A.; Bustamante, M.A.; Churruca, I.; Simon, E. Nutritional differences between a gluten-free diet and a diet containing equivalent products with gluten. *Plant Foods Hum. Nutr.* **2014**, *69*, 182–187. [CrossRef]
45. Vici, G.; Belli, L.; Biondi, M.; Polzonetti, V. Gluten free diet and nutrient deficiencies: A review. *Clin. Nutr.* **2016**, *35*, 1236–1241. [CrossRef] [PubMed]
46. Kulai, T.; Rashid, M. Assessment of Nutritional Adequacy of packaged gluten-free food products. *Can. J. Diet. Pract. Res.* **2014**, *75*, 186–190. [CrossRef] [PubMed]
47. Mazzeo, T.; Cauzzi, S.; Brighenti, F.; Pellegrini, N. The development of a composition database of gluten-free products. *Public Health Nutr.* **2015**, *18*, 1353–1357. [CrossRef]
48. Matos, M.E.; Sanz, T.; Rosell, C.M. Establishing the function of proteins on the rheological and quality properties of rice based gluten free muffins. *Food Hydrocoll.* **2014**, *35*, 150–158. [CrossRef]
49. Cornicelli, M.; Saba, M.; Machello, N.; Silano, M.; Neuhold, S. Nutritional composition of gluten-free food versus regular food sold in the Italian market. *Dig. Liver Dis.* **2018**, *50*, 1305–1308. [CrossRef] [PubMed]
50. Babio, N.; Lladó Bellette, N.; Besora-Moreno, M.; Castillejo, G.; Guillén, N.; Martínez-Cerezo, F.; Vilchez, E.; Roger, E.; Hernández-Alonso, P.; Salas Salvadó, J. A comparison of the nutritional profile and price of gluten-free products and their gluten-containing counterparts available in the Spanish market. *Nutr. Hosp.* **2020**, *37*, 814–822. [CrossRef]
51. Lavriša, Ž.; Hribar, M.; Kušar, A.; Žmitek, K.; Pravst, I. Nutritional composition of gluten-free labelled foods in the Slovenian food supply. *Int. J. Environ. Res. Public Health* **2020**, *17*, 8239. [CrossRef]
52. Roman, L.; Belorio, M.; Gomez, M. Gluten-free breads: The gap between research and commercial reality. *Compr. Rev. Food Sci. Food Saf. (CRFSFS)* **2019**, *18*, 690–702. [CrossRef]
53. Skendi, A.; Papageorgiou, M.; Varzakas, T. High protein substitutes for gluten in gluten-free bread. *Foods* **2021**, *10*, 1997. [CrossRef]
54. Gómez, M. Gluten-free bakery products: Ingredients and processes. *Adv. Food Nutr. Res.* **2022**, *99*, 189–238. [CrossRef] [PubMed]
55. Lasa, A.; Larretxi, I.; Simón, E.; Churruca, I.; Navarro, V.; Martínez, O.; Bustamante, M.; Miranda, J. New software for gluten-free diet evaluation and nutritional education. *Nutrients* **2019**, *11*, 2505. [CrossRef] [PubMed]

56. Šmídová, Z.; Rysová, J. Gluten-free bread and bakery products technology. *Foods* **2022**, *11*, 480. [CrossRef]
57. Graça, C.; Raymundo, A.; Sousa, I. Yogurt and curd cheese as alternative ingredients to improve the gluten-free breadmaking. *Front. Nutr.* **2022**, *9*, 934602. [CrossRef]
58. Monteiro, J.S.; Farage, P.; Zandonadi, R.P.; Botelho, R.B.A.; de Oliveira, L.L.; Raposo, A.; Shakeel, F.; Alshehri, S.; Mahdi, W.A.; Araújo, W.M.C. A systematic review on gluten-free bread formulations using specific volume as a quality indicator. *Foods* **2021**, *10*, 614. [CrossRef] [PubMed]
59. Naqash, F.; Gani, A.; Gani, A.; Masoodi, F.A. Gluten-free baking: Combating the challenges—A review. *Trends Food Sci. Technol.* **2017**, *66*, 98–107. [CrossRef]
60. Taguchi, C.; Kishimoto, Y.; Suzuki-Sugihara, N.; Saita, E.; Usuda, M.; Wang, W.; Masuda, Y.; Kondo, K. Regular egg consumption at breakfast by Japanese woman university students improves daily nutrient intakes: Open-labeled observations. *Asia Pac. J. Clin. Nutr.* **2018**, *27*, 359–365. [CrossRef]
61. Phongthai, S.; D'Amico, S.; Schoenlechner, R.; Rawdkuen, S. Comparative study of rice bran protein concentrate and egg albumin on gluten-free bread properties. *J. Cereal Sci.* **2016**, *72*, 38–45. [CrossRef]
62. Belorio, M.; Sahagún, M.; Gómez, M. Influence of flour particle size distribution on the quality of maize gluten-free cookies. *Foods* **2019**, *8*, 83. [CrossRef]
63. Arslan, M.; Rakha, A.; Xiaobo, Z.; Mahmood, M.A. Complimenting gluten free bakery products with dietary fiber: Opportunities and constraints. *Trends Food Sci. Technol.* **2019**, *83*, 194–202. [CrossRef]
64. Aguiar, E.V.; Santos, F.G.; Centeno, A.; Capriles, V.D. Defining amaranth, buckwheat and quinoa flour levels in gluten-free bread: A simultaneous improvement on physical properties, acceptability and nutrient composition through mixture design. *Foods* **2022**, *11*, 848. [CrossRef] [PubMed]
65. Shepherd, S.J.; Gibson, P.R. Nutritional inadequacies of the gluten-free diet in both recently-diagnosed and long-term patients with coeliac disease. *J. Hum. Nutr. Diet.* **2013**, *26*, 349–358. [CrossRef] [PubMed]
66. Jamieson, J.A.; Gill, K.; Fisher, S.; English, M. Development of a canadian food composition database of gluten-free products. *Foods* **2022**, *11*, 2215. [CrossRef]
67. Duarte, C.; Boccardi, V.; Amaro Andrade, P.; Souza Lopes, A.C.; Jacques, P.F. Dairy versus other saturated fats source and cardiometabolic risk markers: Systematic review of randomized controlled trials. *Crit. Rev. Food Sci. Nutr.* **2021**, *61*, 450–461. [CrossRef]
68. Stantiall, S.E.; Serventi, L. Nutritional and sensory challenges of gluten-free bakery products: A review. *Int. J. Food Sci. Nutr.* **2018**, *69*, 427–436. [CrossRef] [PubMed]
69. Romão, B.; Falcomer, A.L.; Palos, G.; Cavalcante, S.; Botelho, R.B.A.; Nakano, E.Y.; Raposo, A.; Shakeel, F.; Alshehri, S.; Mahdi, W.A.; et al. Glycemic index of gluten-free bread and their main ingredients: A systematic review and meta-analysis. *Foods* **2021**, *10*, 506. [CrossRef]
70. Pacyński, M.; Wojtasiak, R.Z.; Mildner-Szkudlarz, S. Improving the aroma of gluten-free bread. *LWT-Food Sci. Technol.* **2015**, *63*, 706–713. [CrossRef]
71. Tres, A.; Tarnovska, N.; Varona, E.; Quintanilla-Casas, B.; Vichi, S.; Gibert, A.; Vilchez, E.; Guardiola, F. Determination and Comparison of the lipid profile and sodium content of gluten-free and gluten-containing breads from the Spanish market. *Plant Foods Hum. Nutr.* **2020**, *75*, 344–354. [CrossRef]
72. Fry, L.; Madden, A.M.; Fallaize, R. An investigation into the nutritional composition and cost of gluten-free versus regular food products in the UK. *J. Hum. Nutr. Diet.* **2018**, *31*, 108–120. [CrossRef]

nutrients

MDPI

Article

Eating Attitudes of Patients with Celiac Disease in Brazil: A Nationwide Assessment with the EAT-26 Instrument

Luiza Franco [1], Eduardo Yoshio Nakano [2], António Raposo [3,*], Hmidan A. Alturki [4], Sehad N. Alarifi [5], Cláudia Chaves [6], Edite Teixeira-Lemos [7] and Bernardo Romão [1,*]

1 Instituto de Educação Superior de Brasilia, IESB University Center, Brasília 70200-730, Brazil; luizabfranco@gmail.com
2 Department of Statistics, University of Brasília (UnB), Brasília 70910-900, Brazil; eynakano@gmail.com
3 CBIOS (Research Center for Biosciences and Health Technologies), Universidade Lusófona de Humanidades e Tecnologias, Campo Grande 376, 1749-024 Lisboa, Portugal
4 General Directorate for Funds & Grants, King Abdulaziz City for Science & Technology, Riyadh 11442, Saudi Arabia; halturki@kacst.edu.sa
5 Department of Food and Nutrition Science, Al-Quwayiyah College of Sciences and Humanities, Shaqra University, Shaqraa 11971, Saudi Arabia; snalarifi@su.edu.sa
6 ESSV, Centre for Studies in Education and Innovation (CI&DEI), Polytechnic University of Viseu, 3504-510 Viseu, Portugal; claudiachaves21@gmail.com or cchaves@essv.ipv.pt
7 CERNAS Research Centre, Polytechnic University of Viseu, 3504-510 Viseu, Portugal; etlemos3@gmail.com
* Correspondence: antonio.raposo@ulusofona.pt (A.R.); bernardolima156@gmail.com (B.R.)

Abstract: Celiac disease (CD) is an immune-mediated enteropathy triggered by the ingestion of gluten in genetically predisposed individuals. In this sense, a gluten-free diet is the only safe treatment available. Due to the restrictions resulting from this eating pattern, this treatment may impair the relationship of the people with CD with food, increasing the risk of a disordered eating attitude, which is associated with eating disorders. The EAT-26 is a validated instrument already applied worldwide in different populations, and higher scores are suggestive of eating attitudes prone to evolve into eating disorders. Studies carried out in other countries have already shown that people with CD are prone to developing eating disorders; however, no study has been carried out with this theme in the population with CD in Brazil. We carried out a nationwide cross-sectional study in three steps: (i) study design and instrument; (ii) recruitment of participants and ethics; (iii) statistical analysis. A total of 385 participants were included in our sample, 96.36% of them being women. The internal consistency of the applied self-administered Brazilian version of the EAT-26 online questionnaire presented a satisfactory Cronbach's alpha of 0.812, and in total, 36.1% of the respondents were classified with a disordered eating attitude. No differences were found among the scores of participants when divided by categories regarding gender, average monthly income, age, and educational level. However, scores classified as a disordered eating attitude were found in respondents with a body mass index classified as overweight and obese. Our study highlights that disordered eating attitudes are present in overweight and obese women with celiac disease; thus, public health politics are needed to prevent and treat these attitudes.

Keywords: Brazil; celiac disease; eating attitudes; gluten-free diet

1. Introduction

Celiac disease (CD) is an immune-mediated enteropathy triggered by the ingestion of gluten (main protein fraction present in wheat, rye, and barley) in genetically predisposed individuals [1–4]. As for its distribution around the world, studies demonstrate that serological and histological prevalence rates worldwide for the disease are 1.4% and 0.7%, respectively [5]. Clinical signs are broad and may contain typical intestinal features, such as chronic diarrhea, weight loss, and abdominal distention, and atypical recurrent abdominal pain, aphthous stomatitis, short stature, high levels of aminotransferase, fatigue chronic, and reduced bone mineral density, including an iron deficiency with or without anemia [2,6–9]. In addition, CD is associated with an increased prevalence of lymphoproliferative disease, infertility, cancer, and risk of fractures [10–13].

Currently, despite the presence of gluten-specific digestive enzymes on the market, the only safe treatment is the gluten-free diet (GFD); therefore, foods containing this protein fraction should be totally excluded from the diet [1].

The GFD is characterized as a challenging treatment since, in addition to the presence of gluten in traditional food of the Brazilian diet, there is also the risk of the accidental ingestion of this protein fraction through cross-contamination [14,15]. Furthermore, it appears that the cost of these products is higher, and their availability is reduced when compared to their equivalent counterparts that contain gluten [16–18].

Therefore, due to the restrictions arising from this dietary pattern, this treatment may impair the relationship of people with CD with food, increasing the risk of eating disorders [19,20].

Eating disorders (ED) are characterized as abnormal attitudes related to eating or weight control, have a multifactorial etiology, and can be deadly while also considerably impairing the individual's physical health and psychosocial functioning [21–23]. There are several diagnostic methods, such as DSM-5 and ICD-11 [24,25] as well as those that assess attitudes associated with their development, such as the Binge Eating Scale (ECAP), Edinburgh Bulimic Investigation Test (BITE), Restraint Scale, Hay Questionnaire, Eating Attitudes Scale (DEAS), and the Eating Attitudes Test (EAT-26) [26].

EAT-26, in turn, is a 26-item validated instrument that assesses eating attitudes associated with the development of eating disorders, stating that results above the cutoff point suggest higher risk for developing ED [27]. As it is a short, easy-to-apply instrument, it is consolidated as a screening tool for assessing the risk of developing eating disorders in at-risk populations [27].

Studies carried out in other countries have already shown that people with CD are prone to developing EDs. In Italy, a 2013 study indicate that the frequency of altered eating attitude is increased in untreated CD when compared to a control group, with percentage of pathological EAT-26 scores significantly different between groups [28]. In Israel, a 2018 study in adolescents revealed that individuals with CD obtained higher scores on the topics diet, body image, and concern about food [29]. In addition, in the United Kingdom, in 2016, a study showed a higher prevalence of eating disorders assessed with the EAT-26 in celiac disease compared to a healthy control group, with a score of 15.7% above the clinical cutoff point [19].

In this sense, studies regarding dysfunctional eating attitudes among people with CD are needed given that these comorbidities are directly associated with the overall quality of life and the long-term adoption of a GFD [30,31]

However, to date, no study has been carried out in the CD population in Brazil. Therefore, the objective of this study is to analyze the eating attitudes of individuals with celiac disease and relate them to the indication of eating disorders.

2. Materials and Methods

2.1. Study Design and Instrument

A nationwide quantitative cross-sectional study regarding the eating attitudes of patients with CD in Brazil was performed using a validated self-administered instrument (EAT-26), translated to Brazilian Portuguese, and validated [27,32]. A schematic diagram of the study design is available in Figure 1 below.

The EAT-26 questionnaire aims to screen disordered eating attitudes associated with eating disorders and comprises 26 items, with its possible answers distributed among a 6-item Likert-type scale (Always, Usually, Often, Sometimes, Rarely, and Never) [27,32]. Each question is evaluated utilizing a 5-point scale, with "Always" corresponding to 5 points; "Often", 3 points; and "Never", 0 points. In this sense, the maximum punctuation for the questionnaire is 130.

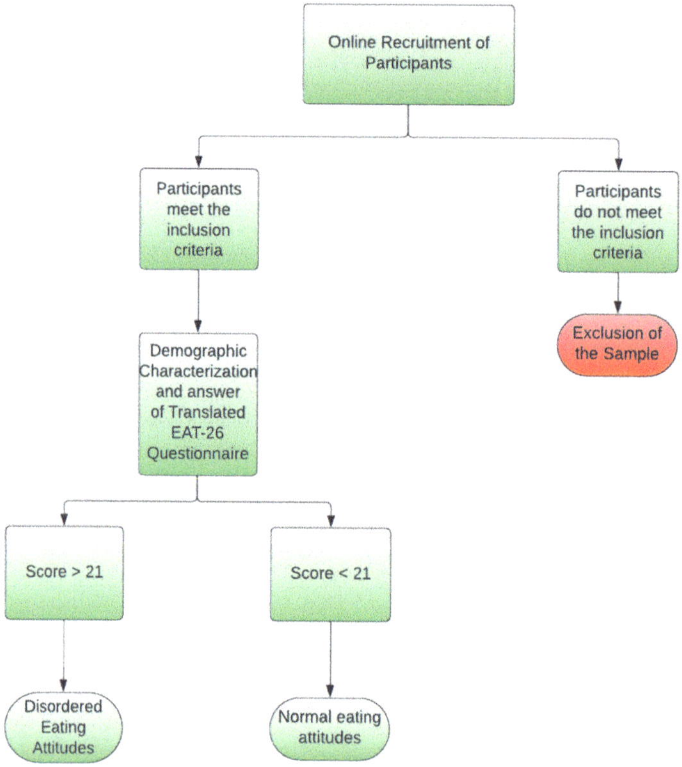

Figure 1. Schematic diagram of the study design.

According to the instrument, participants with scores equal or above 21 were classified with disordered eating attitudes [27,32]. As a part of the EAT-26 questionnaire, self-reported weight and height were also collected, and the respective Body Mass Index (BMI) (kg/m^2) was calculated and classified for each participant according to World Health Organization (WHO) guidelines [33]. The English version of the EAT-26 questionnaire is available in Appendix A.

Besides the Brazilian version of the EAT-26, sociodemographic characteristics previously defined by the Brazilian Institute of Geography and Statistics (IBGE; Instituto Brasileiro de Geografia e Estatística) were also collected, such as gender, place of residency in Brazil, age, average monthly income (BRL), and educational level. For better comprehension of the average monthly income, BRL was converted to USD, utilizing the conversion scale of 1 USD = 4.81 BRL. Google Forms® was used to collect answers of Brazilian patients with CD from 1 May to 1 June 2023.

2.2. Recruitment of Participants and Ethics

The inclusion criteria of participants were (i) to have celiac disease diagnoses for at least two years; (ii) to live in Brazil; (iii) to be at least 18 years of age. Those who did not agree to participate on the research were directed to a page appreciating their time.

The study was approved by the ethics committee of University Center IESB (Instituto de Educação Superior de Brasília) with the registry number CAAE: 69334823.0.0000.8927 and was also conducted according to the Declaration of Helsinki guidelines.

Participants were recruited through artwork posted on social media networks, such as Instagram®, Facebook®, Whatsapp®, and Tik Tok®. In order to obtain a more probative sample of Brazilians with celiac disease, a partnership was signed with the National Federation of Celiac Disease of Brazil (FENACELBRA) and its respective affiliated associations distributed among twenty-six Brazilian states and Federal District (ACELBRAS). Given the low prevalence of celiac disease, a convenience sample was used to determine the number of participants.

2.3. Statistical Analysis

As a resource of Google Forms® platform, all items were mandatory to be completed; in this sense, no missing answers were present. Regarding the internal consistency of the questionnaire, the Cronbach's alpha was calculated with a level of significance of 95% (CI 95%), noting that results equal or above of 0.7 were interpreted as a reliable internal consistency.

Quantitative statistics were presented as their mean and standard deviation. The student's *t*-test and one-way analysis of variance (ANOVA) followed by Tukey's post-hoc test with a significance level of 95% ($p < 0.05$) were performed in order to compare average scores presented by the EAT-26 questionnaire in different stratums, such as BMI (kg/m^2), gender, age, monthly income, and educational level. Software tools Microsoft Excel® (United States, 2023) and IBM SPSS Statistics for Windows (IBM Corp., Armonk, NY, USA, 2023) were used to perform all analyses.

Afterwards, the items were divided according to the EAT-26 scales: Diet Scale (D), Bulimia and Food Preoccupation Scale (B), and Oral Control Scale (OC), then analysis of variance (ANOVA, $p < 0.05$) was applied to statistically compare the scales.

As for the individual analysis of the items in the instrument, first, the total percentages of the answers for each item were grouped. Then, the answers for each item were expressed as percentages of their frequencies. A comparison based on the absolute frequencies between answers of respondents classified with a normal eating attitude and a disordered eating attitude was performed.

3. Results

3.1. Characteristics of the Included Participants

Data collected with the online self-administration of the EAT-26 among Brazilian individuals with CD presented a total response of 394 individuals; however, only 385 participants met the inclusion criteria (>18 years of age), representing in this manner the final sample of the study. The majority of respondents were female (96.36%; $n = 371$), while only 3.37% ($n = 13$) were men. Only one person declared themselves as non-binary (0.25%). A full description of the sociodemographic and BMI data regarding this study's participants is available in Table 1.

Overall, most respondents ($n = 112$; 39.09%) presented an average monthly income of ranging from 5000.01 BRL (USD 1038.71) to 10,000.01 BRL (USD 2077.43), while the minor parcel of respondents ($n = 76$; 19.74%) presented an income of up to 3000.00 BRL (USD 623.00).

Regarding the average age of the respondents, most of our sample comprised people ranging between 25 and 34 years of age ($n = 136$; 35.32%), with people ranging between 18 and 24 years representing the second higher number of participants ($n = 110$; 28.57%). The lower number of participants were above 55 years of age ($n = 2$; 5.19%).

As for the educational level, almost half of the respondents were at the undergraduate level ($n = 189$; 49.09%), while 141 respondents (29.61%) informed us of being at a graduate level or above. Only 14.28% ($n = 55$) of the sample studied until high school only.

Regarding the average BMI of respondents, which was calculated with self-reported weight and height collected through the online questionnaire, most of the sample ($n = 231$; 60%) were classified as normal weight, presenting an average BMI of 17.23 ± 9.13, followed by 21.81% of the sample being classified as overweight (21.44 ± 10.09 Kg/m^2).

A distribution of the place of living among respondents on the five regions of Brazil is disposed as a coropletic map in Figure 2.

Table 1. Sociodemographic and BMI data of the study participants.

Variable	Number	% of the Sample
Gender (F or M)		
Female	371	96.36%
Male	13	3.37%
Average Monthly Income (BRL and USD)		
Up to 3000.00 BRL (USD 623.00)	76	19.94%
3000.01 to 5000 BRL (USD 623.23 to 1038.71)	86	22.33%
5000.01 to 10,000.01 BRL (USD 1038.71 to 2077.43)	112	29.09%
>10,000.01 BRL (USD 2077.43)	111	28.83%
Age (Years)		
18 to 24 years old	110	28.57%
25 to 34 years old	136	35.32%
35 to 44 years old	76	19.74%
45 to 54 years old	43	11.16%
>55 years old	20	5.19%
Educational Level		
Up to High School	55	14.28%
Undergraduate Level (B.Sc)	189	49.09%
Graduate Level or Above (Post-Graduation, Masters degree, or Ph.D.)	141	29.61%
Average BMI (Kg/m^2)		
Underweight (<18.5 Kg/m^2)	18.7 ± 11.29 Kg/m^2; $n = 30$	7.79%
Normal Weight ($\geq$18.5 Kg/m^2 < 25 Kg/m^2)	17.23 ± 9.13 Kg/m^2; $n = 231$	60%
Overweight ($\geq$25 Kg/m^2 < 30 Kg/m^2)	21.44 ± 10.09 Kg/m^2; $n = 84$	21.81%
Obesity ($\geq$30 Kg/m^2)	24.85 ± 11.28 Kg/m^2; $n = 40$	10.38%

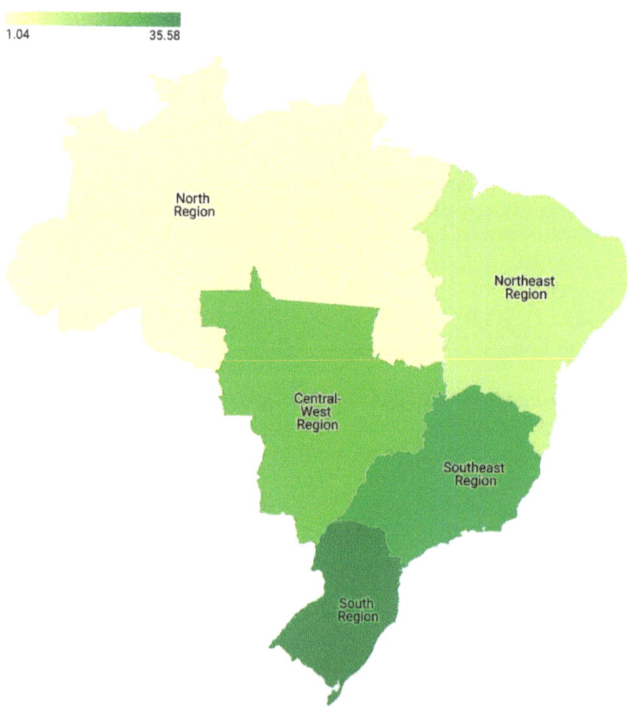

Figure 2. Coropletic map generated from the place of living of respondents in the Brazilian five regions.

In general, most respondents were from the South region (n = 137; 35.85%), followed by 115 respondents residing in the Southeast region (29.87%). The Central–West region contributed 22.86% of the respondents (n = 88), while the Northeast and North regions contributed 10.65% (n = 41) and 1.04% (n = 4), respectively.

3.2. Questionnaire Internal Consistency and Obtained Scores

Among all respondents, 36.1% (n = 139) scored above the cutoff points (>21), resulting in the classification as patients with disordered eating attitudes. Regarding the Cronbach's alpha calculated to evaluate the internal consistency of the questionnaire, the average score of the questionnaire was 19.06 ± 10.06, and the alpha was 0.812 (CI 95%: 0.784–0.838), resulting in a satisfactory internal consistency (>0.7).

As for the average score collected through the online administration of the EAT-26 questionnaire, the scores stratified by sociodemographic variables and average BMI are available in Table 2 below.

Table 2. Average score collected from the self-administered online EAT-26 questionnaire.

Variable	Average Score	p Value
Gender (F or M)		
Female	19.25 ± 10.05 ^{b}	<0.001 *
Male	11.85 ± 3.59 ^{a}	
Average Monthly Income (BRL and USD)		
Up to 3000.00 BRL (USD 623.00)	20.66 ± 11.61 ^{a}	0.355 **
3000.01 to 5000 BRL (USD 623.23 to 1038.71)	17.84 ± 8.57 ^{a}	
5000.01 to 10,000.01 BRL (USD 1038.71 to 2077.43)	18.83 ± 9.39 ^{a}	
>10,000.01 BRL (USD 2077.43)	19.14 ± 10.61 ^{a}	
Age (Years)		
18 to 24 years old	19.19 ± 10.51 ^{a}	0.183 **
25 to 34 years old	19.82 ± 10.82 ^{a}	
35 to 44 years old	16.70 ± 8.60 ^{a}	
45 to 54 years old	20.72 ± 9.78 ^{a}	
>55 years old	18.55 ± 6.47 ^{a}	
Educational Level		
Up to High School	20.02 ± 10.27 ^{b}	0.025 **
Undergraduate Level (B.Sc)	20.14 ± 10.47 ^{b}	
Graduate Level or Above (Post-Graduation, Masters degree, or Ph.D.)	17.23 ± 9.18 ^{a}	
Average Score by BMI (Kg/m^2)		
Underweight (<18.5 Kg/m^2)	18.70 ± 11.23 ^{a}	<0.001 **
Adequate Weight (≥18.5 Kg/m^2 < 25 Kg/m^2)	17.24 ± 9.13 ^{a}	
Overweight (≥25 Kg/m^2 < 30 Kg/m^2)	21.44 ±10.10 ^{ab}	
Obesity (≥30 Kg/m^2)	24.85 ± 11.28 ^{b}	

* Non-paired Student's t-test; ** ANOVA with Tukey's post hoc test. Values in the same category with different superscript letters presented significant differences ($p < 0.05$).

Regarding the gender variable, female respondents presented an average score of 19.25 ± 10.05 points, a higher score in comparison to what is found among male respondents (11.85 ± 3.59). However, none of the groups presented an average score classified as a disordered eating attitude.

As for the average monthly income, no differences were found between all groups of respondents. In addition, no differences were found between respondents among different ages. The educational level seemed to be a determinant factor regarding the obtained scores. Respondents who studied up until high school (20.02 ± 10.27) and obtained an undergraduate degree (20.14 ± 10.47) presented significantly higher scores in comparison to respondents with a graduate degree (17.23 ± 9.18); however, none of the groups were classified with a disordered eating attitude.

Respondents classified both with underweight and adequate weight BMIs did not present significant differences between the obtained scores and did not present a score associated with a disordered eating attitude; nevertheless, overweight and obese respondents presented scores classified as a disordered eating attitude (>21), differing from other groups and presenting higher scores.

The analysis of the questionnaire scales showed that there is no statistically significant difference between their means ($p > 0.05$). This means that we cannot conclude that there are significant differences in respondent scores between the questionnaire's scales.

However, regarding the individual items of the instrument, between the groups with normal (Score < 21) and disordered (Score > 21) eating attitudes, different frequencies for each item were found. Table 3 below presents the frequencies of the answers per item as percentages. A full description of each item is available in Appendix A. Also, the full answer sheet for the collected data is available at Table S1 (Supplementary file).

Table 3. Absolute frequencies of answers per item in the self-administered questionnaire of the groups with normal and disordered eating attitudes.

Item	Always	Usually	Often	Sometimes	Rarely	Never	Always	Usually	Often	Sometimes	Rarely	Never
	Overall Score < 21; Frequency in (%)						Overall Score > 21; Frequency in (%)					
1	10.6	16.3	25.6	12.2	13.8	21.5	25.5	51.8	31.7	9.4	2.2	1.4
2	0.0	1.2	8.1	14.6	28.5	47.6	0.5	1.4	13.7	29.5	9.4	23.0
3	32.5	39.0	15.9	6.1	3.7	2.8	44.4	65.5	23.0	8.6	0.7	1.4
4	1.2	6.1	13.8	19.9	19.1	39.8	10.1	25.9	21.6	18.7	12.2	8.6
5	10.2	17.9	21.1	15.4	16.3	19.1	14.0	20.9	18.0	23.0	16.5	8.6
6	1.6	8.1	14.2	13.0	17.1	45.9	6.2	14.4	24.5	27.3	7.9	12.9
7	2.0	3.3	12.2	14.2	26.4	41.9	2.6	3.6	17.3	33.8	15.8	12.9
8	4.5	7.7	13.0	11.0	18.7	45.1	7.0	11.5	12.2	17.3	12.2	13.7
9	0.0	0.0	0.0	1.2	5.3	93.5	0.0	0.0	2.2	5.0	2.9	9.4
10	0.4	1.6	11.8	13.0	23.2	50.0	6.2	16.5	20.9	25.2	11.5	15.1
11	4.5	8.1	21.1	13.0	16.7	36.6	20.5	48.9	18.7	16.5	2.9	5.0
12	3.7	7.7	18.7	8.5	19.1	42.3	17.4	41.7	17.3	21.6	6.5	5.0
13	5.7	10.2	14.6	15.4	16.7	37.4	6.8	8.6	5.8	15.1	9.4	12.2
14	5.7	11.0	22.4	12.6	23.2	25.2	18.7	41.7	30.2	18.0	2.9	3.6
15	9.3	9.3	19.9	15.0	24.4	22.0	11.7	15.8	17.3	18.7	14.4	15.8
16	2.0	12.6	17.5	18.3	24.4	25.2	4.2	7.9	25.9	24.5	12.9	16.5
17	0.8	3.3	12.2	11.4	26.4	45.9	1.3	2.2	10.8	25.2	10.1	22.3
18	5.3	13.8	17.5	13.8	13.0	36.6	13.2	27.3	25.2	18.7	12.9	7.2
19	22.8	41.5	20.7	8.5	4.5	2.0	19.0	12.2	29.5	28.8	12.2	13.7
20	2.4	3.3	14.6	13.8	24.0	41.9	4.7	8.6	12.9	20.1	12.2	14.4
21	2.4	13.8	21.1	21.5	26.4	14.6	8.1	18.0	30.2	25.9	12.9	7.9
22	0.8	4.1	21.1	15.0	18.3	40.7	4.4	10.8	23.7	28.8	11.5	11.5
23	0.0	2.4	8.5	11.4	19.9	57.7	5.7	15.8	20.9	22.3	11.5	15.8
24	0.0	0.4	6.9	7.7	13.8	71.1	0.8	2.2	15.8	13.7	10.8	17.3
25	3.7	9.8	30.1	21.5	18.3	16.7	5.5	8.6	14.4	27.3	18.0	23.0
26	0.0	1.2	1.6	3.7	7.3	86.2	1.3	3.6	3.6	10.1	5.8	15.1

In general, answers marked as "Always", "Usually", and "Often" are indicative of disordered eating attitudes. As an example, item 1, related to the fear of weight gain due to food intake, was more frequent in the group with scores above 21, and in all items, with the exception of item 19, it was described as "I demonstrate self-control in relation to foods" (Appendix A).

4. Discussion

4.1. Characteristics of the Sample

This is the first study to ever study the presence of disordered eating attitudes among patients with celiac disease (CD) in Brazil. Regarding the final sample, it was noted that it mostly comprised women, similar to other studies conducted in Brazil [30,34].

Although genetic mechanisms are not well defined, it is noteworthy that CD occurs most preeminently in women, with an average ratio of 2.8:1 in relation with men [35]. A recent theory indicates that several factors may contribute to gender differences in autoimmune diseases, such as the exposure to environmental agents; endogenous hormones; differences in biology, such as pregnancy and menstruation; and epigenetic modifications related to chromosomes [36–38]. In addition, a study concluded that female patients with celiac disease carry alterations regarding haplotypes DQ2/DQ8, which are related to the occurrence of celiac disease, more frequently than men [37].

Another possibility is that men tend to obtain a CD diagnosis later than women, given that men also tend to seek less health services compared to women [39,40].

It is also important to highlight that in Brazil's public healthcare, the diagnosis of CD is infrequent or completely unavailable; in this sense, one of the main reflections in the composition of the sample is the number of respondents with an average monthly income above BRL 5000.01 (USD 1038.71) [41,42]. In Brazil, the average household income is BRL 2800.00 (Around USD 582), so it is possible that only the population with higher monthly income has access to diagnostic tests for celiac disease, contributing to the increased share of this population in the included sample [43]. This effect was also noted regarding the place of living of the respondents. In Brazil, the higher gross domestic product (GDP) is concentrated among both South and Southeast regions, both regions with the highest amounts of respondents [43]. However, the increased access to higher education in this parcel of the population might have influenced the increased number of respondents with at least an undergraduate degree [43]. This fact also explains the lower percentage of responses in the North and Northeast regions of Brazil, regions whose GDP is the lowest in the country, possibly reflecting on diagnoses and lines of care in the context of CD.

However, the trend related to the distribution of body composition by income did not follow the pattern observed in the country as a whole. In general, the Brazilian population has a body composition closer to overweight and obese in strata with lower monthly income; on the other hand, more than half of the studied sample presented adequate weight (60%) [44,45].

A possible explanation for this result may be related to the eating attitude of celiac in Brazil. In general, results from research related to the overall quality of life of celiac demonstrate that Brazilian celiac have good results regarding the understanding of the disease and the quality of the diet necessary to control it [30,34,42].

4.2. Scores Obtained from the Self-Administered Online Questionnaire

In our sample, we reached only 13 responses from men, and none obtained a score greater than 21, demonstrating no disordered eating attitudes associated with an eating disorder [32]. There are few studies on disordered attitudes in men only, as there is a persistent view over time that eating disorders are linked to the female gender, which led to an underestimation of disordered eating attitudes and eating disorders in men [46,47]. It is notable in the studies regarding disordered eating attitudes that most of them have small clinical samples, the frequent use of diagnosis tools adapted for women, and especially the discomfort of male patients in resorting to services that are aimed mainly at women, as it is the case in Eds [48].

Gender differences reported within the literature depend on the specific symptoms of the eating disorder. Girls or women are more likely than boys or men to report weight dissatisfaction, dieting for weight control, and purge use, but they are just as likely or less likely than boys or men to report binge eating and use excessive exercise for weight control [49,50]. However, it has been shown that women are more likely than men to report body-checking attitudes, such as ritualistic weighing or trying on special clothing to check how it fits [47].

Regarding the included sample, when separating the participants by age, average monthly income, and educational level, it was noted that scores classified as disordered eating attitudes were not obtained; nevertheless, respondents with an educational level of high school or with an undergraduate degree presented higher scores in comparison to participants with at least a graduate-level degree.

In general, lower levels of education (below high school) are already associated with risk factors for the development of eating disorders, with the main theory being the fact that, associated with lower education, there is also evidence of lower monthly income and impaired access to health services [51,52].

However, some studies show that an undergraduate degree obtained from college courses negatively influence stress and mental health in general in groups of people with adequate weight and who are overweight and obese, thus increasing the risk of developing eating disorders [53,54]. In this sense, although the scores obtained are not sufficient to be considered associated with disordered eating attitudes, it is important to emphasize that the mentioned groups are at greater risk compared to the group of graduates in addition to the score being close to the point cutting stipulated by the instrument [27,32].

However, a critical point verified from the analyses is related to the BMI of the participants. In our research, overweight and obese participants presented scores classified as a disordered eating attitude (>21), with significantly higher scores in comparison to the remaining groups. Concern about weight is a common constant within the biopsychosocial process of developing eating disorders [55]; in addition, in our study, a considerable number of respondents referred to being constantly worried about gaining weight (Table 3). Frequently and more prominently in women, studies report social pressures related to the presented body composition, with individuals reporting impaired mental health, self-esteem, reduced job opportunities, social life, and difficulties in relationships [54,56].

In this sense, the occurrence of disordered eating attitudes increases since they appear as a "quick" alternative to obtain weight loss and satisfactory aesthetic results [57]. Although it is important to highlight that in addition to these attitudes being unhealthy, they very commonly produce effects contrary to the desired, contributing as an important risk factor in the increase in the prevalence of being overweight and obese [53,56,57].

As a fact, studies demonstrate that eating disorders, such as binge eating disorder (BED) and strict dieting, are common antecedents in obese women, thus supporting the results found among our sample [58–61]. Regarding items related to BED in the applied instrument, it was noted that the response frequency to item 25 (I like to try new high-calorie foods) was higher in the population with the highest score on the instrument, suggesting a critical point of risk.

In comparison with other studies conducted in Brazil that used the same instrument but in populations of women without celiac disease, the results showed frequencies of disordered eating attitudes varying between 16.5% and 30.1%, with no differences between different body mass indexes among respondents [52,62]. In this sense, our study presented a higher frequency for disordered eating attitudes, supporting our hypothesis that patients with celiac disease are more prone to develop this kind of issue given the nature of the restrictive treatment. However, more studies comparing populations with and without celiac disease are needed to better support this theory.

In celiac disease specifically, studies performed in other countries already show a higher prevalence of disordered eating attitudes compared to the general population, both among men and women [29].

A theory is that, with this condition, patients often a need to monitor the gluten content of foods along with fears about the effectiveness of the diet and concerns about preventing symptoms [63–65]. A point that corroborates this theory is the frequency of "Always" answers to question 3 (I feel worried about food) and the frequency of "Often" to question 19 (I demonstrate self-control in relation to food) of the applied questionnaire

(Table 3), which relates with the constant concern with food, suggesting a critical attitude point within the Brazilian celiac community.

In addition, it is noticeable that untreated gastrointestinal symptoms can trigger an aversion to food, which can influence disordered attitudes and attitude [19]. The Satherley, Higgs, and Howard (2017) theoretical model suggests two pathways of eating disorders in gastrointestinal diseases, one of which is the post-diagnosis weight gain experiment [66]. This can also be demonstrated in the higher frequency of answers (always, often, and sometimes) to question 1 (I am terrified with the idea of getting fat) and 14 (I am worried about the idea of having fat in my body) of the applied questionnaire (Table 3).

People affected with gastrointestinal diseases, such as the celiac disease, may believe that their diet causes them to gain weight, which leads to dysfunctional diet beliefs and attitudes, such as a lack of adherence to the dietary regimen, ongoing gastrointestinal symptoms, and psychological distress [67]. In the literature, there is a study that describes three cases in which the concern with weight increased after starting a gluten-free diet [68].

Indeed, such a theory is supported by the nutritional quality of commercial gluten-free foods. In general, it is noted that gluten-free foods often use high-glycemic index flours, with a high carbohydrate content and less dietary fiber compared to their gluten-containing counterparts [69–71]. In addition, a higher energy content is evident given that, often, a higher quantity of fat is implemented as an ingredient to improve sensory and technological characteristics of gluten-free products [72].

In this sense, the adoption of public policies stands out, both with regard to access to healthier gluten-free products and the creation of policies that seek to prevent and treat disordered eating attitudes associated with eating disorders in people with celiac disease in Brazil.

Regarding the limitations of this study, it is important to highlight that the instrument did not assess whether the participants were following a strictly gluten-free diet. Furthermore, the presence of other comorbidities that require attention to nutrition, such as Type 1 diabetes mellitus, was not assessed in this study and may therefore have influenced a small portion of respondents given the concomitant occurrence of this disease with CD. In addition, although disordered eating attitudes are associated with a greater risk of developing eating disorders, our study did not utilize instruments for the diagnosis of any eating disorder.

5. Conclusions

In conclusion, we believe that our study brings together an important research area for the first time in Brazil. A total of 36.1% of the included sample presented scores classified as a disordered eating attitude; however, the stratification of the data showed that women with celiac disease and BMIs classified as overweight and obese presented higher scores in comparison to other sociodemographic characteristics. It is important to note that disordered eating attitudes are associated with a higher risk of developing eating disorders; thus, our study highlights the need for the implementation of public health policies directed to this public in order to prevent and treat those disordered eating attitudes.

Supplementary Materials: The following supporting information can be downloaded at: https://www.mdpi.com/article/10.3390/nu15224796/s1, Table S1: Full data collected from the self-administered translated to Brazilian Portuguese version of the EAT-26 questionnaire.

Author Contributions: Conceptualization, L.F. and B.R.; methodology, B.R.; software, E.Y.N. and B.R.; validation, B.R.; formal analysis, L.F. and B.R.; investigation, L.F. and B.R.; resources, B.R; data curation, L.F., B.R. and E.Y.N.; writing—original draft preparation, L.F.; writing—review and editing, A.R., H.A.A., S.N.A., C.C., E.T.-L. and B.R.; visualization, A.R. and B.R.; supervision, A.R. and B.R.; project administration, A.R. and B.R.; funding acquisition, A.R., C.C., E.T.-L. and B.R. All authors have read and agreed to the published version of the manuscript.

Funding: This work is funded by National Funds through the FCT-Foundation for Science and Technology, I.P., within the scope of the projects Refª UIDB/05507/2020 and UIDB/00681/202.

Institutional Review Board Statement: The study was approved by the ethics committee of University Center IESB (Instituto de Educação Superior de Brasília) with the registry number CAAE: 69334823.0.0000.8927 and was also conducted according to the Declaration of Helsinki guidelines.

Informed Consent Statement: Informed consent was obtained from all subjects involved in the study.

Data Availability Statement: Data are contained within the article and supplementary materials.

Acknowledgments: This work was supported by the FCT—Foundation for Science and Technology, Portugal. Furthermore, we would like to thank the Centre for Studies in Education and Innovation (CI&DEI), Centre for Natural Resources, Environment and Society (CERNAS) and the Institute Polytechnic of Viseu for their support.

Conflicts of Interest: The authors declare no conflict of interest.

Appendix A

Validated Version of the EAT-26 questionnaire [27].
Name:____
Age:______ Weight:______ Height:_____

Please Answer All the Following Items	Always	Usually	Often	Sometimes	Rarely	Never
1—I'm terrified of the idea of gaining weight						
2—I avoid eating when I'm hungry						
3—I feel worried about food						
4—Continuing to overeat makes me feel like I can't stop						
5—I cut my food into small pieces						
6—I pay attention to the number of calories in the food I eat						
7—I particularly avoid foods rich in carbohydrates (e.g., bread, rice, potatoes, etc.)						
8—I feel like others would like me to eat more.						
9—Vomiting after eating						
10—I feel extremely guilty after eating						
11—I worry about wanting to be thinner						
12—I think about burning extra calories when I exercise						
13—People think I'm too thin						
14—I worry about having fat on my body						
15—It takes me longer to eat my meals than other people						
16—I avoid eating foods that contain sugar						
17—I usually eat diet foods						
18—I feel like food controls my life						
19—I demonstrate self-control around food						
20—I feel like others pressure me to eat						
21—I spend a lot of time thinking about eating						
22—I feel discomfort after eating sweets						
23—I follow weight loss regimes						
24—I like feeling my stomach empty						
25—I like to try new high-calorie foods						
26—I feel like vomiting after meals						

References

1. Catassi, C.; Fasano, A. Celiac Disease. *Curr. Opin. Gastroenterol.* **2008**, *24*, 687–691. [CrossRef]
2. Di Sabatino, A.; Corazza, G.R. Coeliac Disease. *Lancet* **2009**, *373*, 1480–1493. [CrossRef]
3. Ludvigsson, J.F.; Bai, J.C.; Biagi, F.; Card, T.R.; Ciacci, C.; Ciclitira, P.J.; Green, P.H.R.; Hadjivassiliou, M.; Holdoway, A.; van Heel, D.A.; et al. Diagnosis and Management of Adult Coeliac Disease: Guidelines from the British Society of Gastroenterology. *Gut* **2014**, *63*, 1210–1228. [CrossRef]
4. Leffler, D.; Saha, S.; Farrell, R.J. Celiac Disease. *Am. J. Manag. Care* **2003**, *9*, 825–883. [PubMed]
5. Singh, P.; Arora, A.; Strand, T.A.; Leffler, D.A.; Catassi, C.; Green, P.H.; Kelly, C.P.; Ahuja, V.; Makharia, G.K. Global Prevalence of Celiac Disease: Systematic Review and Meta-Analysis. *Clin. Gastroenterol. Hepatol.* **2018**, *16*, 823–836. [CrossRef] [PubMed]

6. Fasano, A.; Catassi, C. Celiac Disease. *N. Engl. J. Med.* **2012**, *367*, 2419–2426. [CrossRef] [PubMed]
7. Groll, A. Short Stature as the Primary Manifestation of Coeliac Disease. *Lancet* **1980**, *316*, 1097–1099. [CrossRef] [PubMed]
8. Bergamaschi, G.; Markopoulos, K.; Albertini, R.; Di Sabatino, A.; Biagi, F.; Ciccocioppo, R.; Arbustini, E.; Corazza, G.R. Anemia of Chronic Disease and Defective Erythropoietin Production in Patients with Celiac Disease. *Haematologica* **2008**, *93*, 1785–1791. [CrossRef] [PubMed]
9. Biel, K.; Böhm, M.; Luger, T.A.; Bonsmann, G. Long-Standing Oral Aphthae—A Clue to the Diagnosis of Coeliac Disease. *Dermatology* **2000**, *200*, 340. [CrossRef]
10. Ludvigsson, J.; Montgomery, S.; Ekbom, A. Celiac Disease and Risk of Adverse Fetal Outcome: A Population-Based Cohort Study. *Gastroenterology* **2005**, *129*, 454–463. [CrossRef]
11. West, J.; Logan, R.F.A.; Smith, C.J.; Hubbard, R.B.; Card, T.R. Malignancy and Mortality in People with Coeliac Disease: Population Based Cohort Study. *BMJ* **2004**, *329*, 716–719. [CrossRef] [PubMed]
12. West, J.; Logan, R.F.A.; Card, T.R.; Smith, C.; Hubbard, R. Fracture Risk in People with Celiac Disease: A Population-Based Cohort Study. *Gastroenterology* **2003**, *125*, 429–436. [CrossRef] [PubMed]
13. Pelizzaro, F.; Marsilio, I.; Fassan, M.; Piazza, F.; Barberio, B.; D'Odorico, A.; Savarino, E.V.; Farinati, F.; Zingone, F. The Risk of Malignancies in Celiac Disease—A Literature Review. *Cancers* **2021**, *13*, 5288. [CrossRef] [PubMed]
14. Farage, P.; Zandonadi, R.P.; Gandolfi, L.; Pratesi, R.; Falcomer, A.L.; Araújo, L.S.; Nakano, E.Y.; Ginani, V.C. Accidental Gluten Contamination in Traditional Lunch Meals from Food Services in Brasilia, Brazil. *Nutrients* **2019**, *11*, 1924. [CrossRef]
15. Falcomer, A.L.; Santos Araújo, L.; Farage, P.; Santos Monteiro, J.; Yoshio Nakano, E.; Puppin Zandonadi, R. Gluten Contamination in Food Services and Industry: A Systematic Review. *Crit. Rev. Food Sci. Nutr.* **2020**, *60*, 479–493. [CrossRef]
16. Alencar, N.M.M.; Araújo, V.A.; Faggian, L.; Silveira Araújo, M.B.; Capriles, V.D. What about Gluten-free Products? An Insight on Celiac Consumers' Opinions and Expectations. *J. Sens. Stud.* **2021**, *36*, e12664. [CrossRef]
17. Bagolin do Nascimento, A.; Medeiros Rataichesck Fiates, G.; dos Anjos, A.; Teixeira, E. Availability, Cost and Nutritional Composition of Gluten-Free Products. *Br. Food J.* **2014**, *116*, 1842–1852. [CrossRef]
18. da Silva, L.A.; Tavares, I.M.d.C.; de Oliveira, C.P.; de Oliveira, J.R.; Irfan, M.; Bilal, M.; Franco, M. Nutritional Quality and Price of Regular Food versus Gluten-Free on E-Commerce Platforms. *Res. Soc. Dev.* **2021**, *10*, e137101018751. [CrossRef]
19. Satherley, R.-M.; Howard, R.; Higgs, S. The Prevalence and Predictors of Disordered Eating in Women with Coeliac Disease. *Appetite* **2016**, *107*, 260–267. [CrossRef]
20. Whitaker, J.K.H.; West, J.; Holmes, G.K.T.; Logan, R.F.A. Patient Perceptions of the Burden of Coeliac Disease and Its Treatment in the UK. *Aliment. Pharmacol. Ther.* **2009**, *29*, 1131–1136. [CrossRef]
21. Treasure, J.; Duarte, T.A.; Schmidt, U. Eating Disorders. *Lancet* **2020**, *395*, 899–911. [CrossRef] [PubMed]
22. Nunes, L.G.; Santos, M.C.S.; Souza, A.A. Fatores de Risco Associados Ao Desenvolvimento de Bulimia e Anorexia Nervosa Em Estudantes Universitários: Uma Revisão Integrativa. *HU Rev.* **2017**, *43*, 1–13. [CrossRef]
23. Galmiche, M.; Déchelotte, P.; Lambert, G.; Tavolacci, M.P. Prevalence of Eating Disorders over the 2000–2018 Period: A Systematic Literature Review. *Am. J. Clin. Nutr.* **2019**, *109*, 1402–1413. [CrossRef]
24. Moreira-Almeida, A.; Cardeña, E. Diagnóstico Diferencial Entre Experiências Espirituais e Psicóticas Não Patológicas e Transtornos Mentais: Uma Contribuição de Estudos Latino-Americanos Para o CID-11. *Rev. Bras. Psiquiatr.* **2011**, *33*, s21–s28. [CrossRef]
25. Araújo, Á.C.; Neto, F.L. A Nova Classificação Americana Para Os Transtornos Mentais—O DSM-5. *Rev. Bras. Ter. Comport. E Cogn.* **2014**, *16*, 67–82. [CrossRef]
26. Freitas, S.; Gorenstein, C.; Appolinario, J.C. Instrumentos Para a Avaliação Dos Transtornos Alimentares. *Rev. Bras. Psiquiatr.* **2002**, *24*, 34–38. [CrossRef]
27. Bighetti, F.; Dos Santos, C.B.; Dos Santos, J.E.; Pilot Pessa, R. Translation and Validation of the Eating Attitudes Test in Female Adolescents in Ribeirão Preto, SP, Brazil. *J. Bras. Psiquiatr.* **2004**, *53*, 339–346.
28. Passananti, V.; Siniscalchi, M.; Zingone, F.; Bucci, C.; Tortora, R.; Iovino, P.; Ciacci, C. Prevalence of Eating Disorders in Adults with Celiac Disease. *Gastroenterol. Res. Pract.* **2013**, *2013*, 491657. [CrossRef]
29. Tokatly Latzer, I.; Lerner-Geva, L.; Stein, D.; Weiss, B.; Pinhas-Hamiel, O. Disordered Eating Behaviors in Adolescents with Celiac Disease. *Eat. Weight. Disord.—Stud. Anorex. Bulim. Obes.* **2020**, *25*, 365–371. [CrossRef]
30. Pratesi, C.P.; Häuser, W.; Uenishi, R.H.; Selleski, N.; Nakano, E.Y.; Gandolfi, L.; Pratesi, R.; Zandonadi, R.P. Quality of Life of Celiac Patients in Brazil: Questionnaire Translation, Cultural Adaptation and Validation. *Nutrients* **2018**, *10*, 1167. [CrossRef]
31. White, L.E.; Bannerman, E.; Gillett, P.M. Coeliac Disease and the Gluten-Free Diet: A Review of the Burdens; Factors Associated with Adherence and Impact on Health-Related Quality of Life, with Specific Focus on Adolescence. *J. Hum. Nutr. Diet.* **2016**, *29*, 593–606. [CrossRef] [PubMed]
32. Garner, D.M.; Bohr, Y.; Garfinkel, P.E. The Eating Attitudes Test: Psychometric Features and Clinical Correlates. *Psychol. Med.* **1982**, *12*, 871–878. [CrossRef] [PubMed]
33. Duggan, M.B. Anthropometry as a Tool for Measuring Malnutrition: Impact of the New WHO Growth Standards and Reference. *Int. Child Health* **2013**, *30*, 1–17. [CrossRef] [PubMed]
34. Falcomer, A.L.; Farage, P.; Pratesi, C.B.; Pratesi, R.; Gandolfi, L.; Nakano, E.Y.; Raposo, A.; Zandonadi, R.P. Health-Related Quality of Life and Experiences of Brazilian Celiac Individuals over the Course of the SARS-CoV-2 Pandemic. *Nutrients* **2021**, *13*, 1582. [CrossRef]

35. Thomas, H.J.; Ahmad, T.; Rajaguru, C.; Barnardo, M.; Warren, B.F.; Jewell, D.P. Contribution of Histological, Serological, and Genetic Factors to the Clinical Heterogeneity of Adult-Onset Coeliac Disease. *Scand. J. Gastroenterol.* **2009**, *44*, 1076–1083. [CrossRef]
36. Ngo, S.T.; Steyn, F.J.; McCombe, P.A. Gender Differences in Autoimmune Disease. *Front. Neuroendocrinol.* **2014**, *35*, 347–369. [CrossRef]
37. Megiorni, F.; Mora, B.; Bonamico, M.; Barbato, M.; Montuori, M.; Viola, F.; Trabace, S.; Mazzilli, M.C. HLA-DQ and Susceptibility to Celiac Disease: Evidence for Gender Differences and Parent-of-Origin Effects. *Am. J. Gastroenterol.* **2008**, *103*, 997–1003. [CrossRef]
38. Jansson-Knodell, C.L.; King, K.S.; Larson, J.J.; Van Dyke, C.T.; Murray, J.A.; Rubio-Tapia, A. Gender-Based Differences in a Population-Based Cohort with Celiac Disease: More Alike than Unalike. *Dig. Dis. Sci.* **2018**, *63*, 184–192. [CrossRef]
39. Pinkhasov, R.M.; Wong, J.; Kashanian, J.; Lee, M.; Samadi, D.B.; Pinkhasov, M.M.; Shabsigh, R. Are Men Shortchanged on Health? Perspective on Health Care Utilization and Health Risk Behavior in Men and Women in the United States. *Int. J. Clin. Pract.* **2010**, *64*, 475–487. [CrossRef]
40. Singh, P.; Arora, S.; Singh, A.; Strand, T.A.; Makharia, G.K. Prevalence of Celiac Disease in Asia: A Systematic Review and Meta-Analysis. *J. Gastroenterol. Hepatol.* **2016**, *31*, 1095–1101. [CrossRef]
41. Pratesi, R.; Gandolfi, L. Doença Celíaca: A Afecção Com Múltiplas Faces Celiac Disease: A Disease with Many Faces. *J. Pediatr. Rio. J.* **2005**, *81*, 357–358. [CrossRef]
42. Machado, J.; Gandolfi, L.; Coutinho De Almeida, F.; Malta Almeida, L.; Puppin Zandonadi, R.; Pratesi, R. Gluten-Free Dietary Compliance in Brazilian Celiac Patients: Questionnaire versus Serological Test. *Nutr. Clin. Y Diet. Hosp.* **2013**, *33*, 46–49. [CrossRef]
43. Instituto Brasileiro de Geografia e Estatística. *Pesquisa Nacional Por Amostra de Domicílio*; Instituto Brasileiro de Geografia e Estatística: Brasília, Brazil, 2023; pp. 1–230.
44. da Costa Louzada, M.L.; Baraldi, L.G.; Steele, E.M.; Martins, A.P.B.; Canella, D.S.; Moubarac, J.C.; Levy, R.B.; Cannon, G.; Afshin, A.; Imamura, F.; et al. Consumption of Ultra-Processed Foods and Obesity in Brazilian Adolescents and Adults. *Prev. Med. Baltim* **2015**, *81*, 9–15. [CrossRef] [PubMed]
45. Leite Canhada, S.; Cristine Luft, V.; Giatti, L.; Bartholow Duncan, B.; Chor, D.; de Jesus da Fonseca, M.M.; Maria Alvim Matos, S.; del Carmen Bisi Molina, M.; Maria Barreto, S.; Bertazzi Levy, R.; et al. Ultra-Processed Foods, Incident Overweight and Obesity, and Longitudinal Changes in Weight and Waist Circumference: The Brazilian Longitudinal Study of Adult Health (ELSA-Brasil). *Public Health Nutr.* **2019**, *23*, 1076–1086. [CrossRef] [PubMed]
46. Striegel-Moore, R.H.; Bulik, C.M. Risk Factors for Eating Disorders. *Am. Psychol.* **2007**, *62*, 181–198. [CrossRef]
47. Striegel-Moore, R.H.; Rosselli, F.; Perrin, N.; DeBar, L.; Wilson, G.T.; May, A.; Kraemer, H.C. Gender Difference in the Prevalence of Eating Disorder Symptoms. *Int. J. Eat. Disord.* **2009**, *42*, 471–474. [CrossRef]
48. Manzato, E. Eating Disorders and Disordered Eating Behaviors in Males: A Challenging Topic. *Eat. Weight. Disord. —Stud. Anorex. Bulim. Obes.* **2019**, *24*, 651–652. [CrossRef] [PubMed]
49. Anderson, C.B.; Bulik, C.M. Gender Differences in Compensatory Behaviors, Weight and Shape Salience, and Drive for Thinness. *Eat. Behav.* **2004**, *5*, 1–11. [CrossRef] [PubMed]
50. Lewinsohn, P.M.; Seeley, J.R.; Moerk, K.C.; Striegel-Moore, R.H. Gender Differences in Eating Disorder Symptoms in Young Adults. *Int. J. Eat. Disord.* **2002**, *32*, 426–440. [CrossRef] [PubMed]
51. Mulders-Jones, B.; Mitchison, D.; Girosi, F.; Hay, P. Socioeconomic Correlates of Eating Disorder Symptoms in an Australian Population-Based Sample. *PloS ONE* **2017**, *12*, e0170603. [CrossRef]
52. Alvarenga, M.d.S.; Scagliusi, F.B.; Philippi, S.T. Comportamento de Risco Para Transtorno Alimentar Em Universitárias Brasileiras. *Arch. Clin. Psychiatry* **2011**, *38*, 03–07. [CrossRef]
53. Mitchell, J.E.; King, W.C.; Courcoulas, A.; Dakin, G.; Elder, K.; Engel, S.; Flum, D.; Kalarchian, M.; Khandelwal, S.; Pender, J.; et al. Eating Behavior and Eating Disorders in Adults before Bariatric Surgery. *Int. J. Eat. Disord.* **2015**, *48*, 215–222. [CrossRef] [PubMed]
54. Pinaquy, S.; Chabrol, H.; Simon, C.; Louvet, J.P.; Barbe, P. Emotional Eating, Alexithymia, and Binge-Eating Disorder in Obese Women. *Obes. Res.* **2003**, *11*, 195–201. [CrossRef] [PubMed]
55. Hrabosky, J.I.; Masheb, R.M.; White, M.A.; Grilo, C.M. Overvaluation of Shape and Weight in Binge Eating Disorder. *J. Consult. Clin. Psychol.* **2007**, *75*, 175–180. [CrossRef]
56. McCuen-Wurst, C.; Ruggieri, M.; Allison, K.C. Disordered Eating and Obesity: Associations between Binge-Eating Disorder, Night-Eating Syndrome, and Weight-Related Comorbidities. *Ann. N. Y. Acad. Sci.* **2018**, *1411*, 96–105. [CrossRef]
57. Gowers, S.G.; Shore, A. Development of Weight and Shape Concerns in the Aetiology of Eating Disorders. *Br. J. Psychiatry* **2001**, *179*, 236–242. [CrossRef]
58. Wadden, T.A.; Foster, G.D.; Sarwer, D.B.; Anderson, D.A.; Gladis, M.; Sanderson, R.S.; Letchak, R.V.; Berkowitz, R.I.; Phelan, S. Dieting and the Development of Eating Disorders in Obese Women: Results of a Randomized Controlled Trial. *Am. J. Clin. Nutr.* **2004**, *80*, 560–568. [CrossRef]
59. Fassino, S.; Leombruni, P.; Pierò, A.; Abbate-Daga, G.; Rovera, G.G. Mood, Eating Attitudes, and Anger in Obese Women with and without Binge Eating Disorder. *J. Psychosom. Res.* **2003**, *54*, 559–566. [CrossRef]

60. Greeno, C.G.; Wing, R.R.; Shiffman, S. Binge Antecedents in Obese Women with and without Binge Eating Disorder. *J. Consult. Clin. Psychol.* **2000**, *68*, 95–102. [CrossRef]
61. Specker, S.; de Zwaan, M.; Raymond, N.; Mitchell, J. Psychopathology in Subgroups of Obese Women with and without Binge Eating Disorder. *Compr. Psychiatry* **1994**, *35*, 185–190. [CrossRef]
62. Nunes, M.A.; Barras, F.C.; Anselmo Olinto, M.T.; Carney, S.; Mari, J.D.J. Prevalence of Abnormal Eating Behaviours and Inappropriate Methods of Weight Control in Young Women from Brazil: A Population-Based Study. *Eat. Weight. Disord.* **2003**, *8*, 100–106. [CrossRef] [PubMed]
63. Ciacci, C.; Zingone, F. The Perceived Social Burden in Celiac Disease. *Diseases* **2015**, *3*, 102–110. [CrossRef] [PubMed]
64. Zarkadas, M.; Dubois, S.; MacIsaac, K.; Cantin, I.; Rashid, M.; Roberts, K.C.; La Vieille, S.; Godefroy, S.; Pulido, O.M. Living with Coeliac Disease and a Gluten-Free Diet: A Canadian Perspective. *J. Hum. Nutr. Diet.* **2013**, *26*, 10–23. [CrossRef] [PubMed]
65. Gholmie, Y.; Lee, A.R.; Satherley, R.-M.; Schebendach, J.; Zybert, P.; Green, P.H.R.; Lebwohl, B.; Wolf, R. Maladaptive Food Attitudes and Behaviors in Individuals with Celiac Disease and Their Association with Quality of Life. *Dig. Dis. Sci.* **2023**, *68*, 2899–2907. [CrossRef]
66. Satherley, R.-M.; Higgs, S.; Howard, R. Disordered Eating Patterns in Coeliac Disease: A Framework Analysis. *J. Hum. Nutr. Diet.* **2017**, *30*, 724–736. [CrossRef]
67. Satherley, R.; Howard, R.; Higgs, S. Disordered Eating Practices in Gastrointestinal Disorders. *Appetite* **2015**, *84*, 240–250. [CrossRef]
68. Leffler, D.A.; Dennis, M.; Edwards George, J.B.; Kelly, C.P. The Interaction between Eating Disorders and Celiac Disease: An Exploration of 10 Cases. *Eur. J. Gastroenterol. Hepatol.* **2007**, *19*, 251–255. [CrossRef]
69. Romão, B.; Falcomer, A.L.; Palos, G.; Cavalcante, S.; Braz, R.; Botelho, A.; Nakano, E.Y.; Raposo, A.; Shakeel, F.; Alshehri, S.; et al. Glycemic Index of Gluten-Free Bread and Their Main Ingredients: A Systematic Review and Meta-Analysis. *Foods* **2021**, *10*, 506. [CrossRef]
70. Calvo-Lerma, J.; Crespo-Escobar, P.; Martínez-Barona, S.; Fornés-Ferrer, V.; Donat, E.; Ribes-Koninckx, C. Differences in the Macronutrient and Dietary Fibre Profile of Gluten-Free Products as Compared to Their Gluten-Containing Counterparts. *Eur. J. Clin. Nutr.* **2019**, *73*, 930–936. [CrossRef]
71. Do Nascimento, A.B.; Fiates, G.M.R.; Dos Anjos, A.; Teixeira, E. Analysis of Ingredient Lists of Commercially Available Gluten-Free and Gluten-Containing Food Products Using the Text Mining Technique. *Int. J. Food Sci. Nutr.* **2013**, *64*, 217–222. [CrossRef]
72. Romão, B.; Botelho, R.B.A.; Alencar, E.R.; da Silva, V.S.N.; Pacheco, M.T.B.; Zandonadi, R.P. Chemical Composition and Glycemic Index of Gluten-Free Bread Commercialized in Brazil. *Nutrients* **2020**, *12*, 2234. [CrossRef] [PubMed]

nutrients

MDPI

Article

From Struggle to Strength: A Multicentric Study on How Public Policies for Celiac Disease Transform Lives

Ana Luísa Falcomer [1,*], Claudia B. Pratesi [2,*], Eduardo Yoshio Nakano [3], Cláudia Chaves [4], Mohammad Rostami-Nejad [5], Morad Guennouni [6,7], Ayşegül Aksan [8], Jacques Pouchot [9], Winfried Häuser [10] and Renata Puppin Zandonadi [1,*]

1 Department of Nutrition, School of Health Sciences, University of Brasilia, Brasilia 70910-900, Brazil
2 College of Population Health, University of New Mexico, Albuquerque, NM 87131, USA
3 Department of Statistics, University of Brasilia, Brasilia 70910-900, Brazil; nakano@unb.br
4 ESSV, Centre for Studies in Education and Innovation (CI&DEI), Polytechnic University of Viseu, 3504-510 Viseu, Portugal; cchaves@essv.ipv.pt
5 Celiac Disease and Gluten Related Disorders Research Center, Research Institute for Gastroenterology and Liver Diseases, Shahid Beheshti University of Medical Sciences, Tehran 1416634793, Iran; m.rostamii@gmail.com
6 Science and Technology Team, Higher School of Education and Training, Chouaib Doukkali University of El Jadida, El Jadida 24000, Morocco; morad.guennouni@gmail.com
7 Laboratory of Health Sciences and Technologies, Higher Institute of Health Sciences of Settat, Hassan First University of Settat, Settat 26000, Morocco
8 Institute of Nutritional Science, Justus-Liebig University, 35392 Giessen, Germany; ayseguel.aksan@ernaehrung.uni-giessen.de
9 Service de Médecine Interne, Hôpital Européen Georges Pompidou, Assistance Publique–Hôpitaux de Paris, Université Paris Cité, 75015 Paris, France; jacques.pouchot@egp.aphp.fr
10 Medizinisches Versorgungszentrum für Schmerzmedizin und Seelische Gesundheit Saarbrücken—St. Johann Health Care Center Pain Medicine and Mental Health Saarbrücken, St. Johann Großherzog-Friedrich-Straße 44, 66111 Saarbrücken, Germany; winfriedhaeuser@googlemail.com
* Correspondence: anafalcomer@gmail.com (A.L.F.); cbpratesi@salud.unm.edu (C.B.P.); renatapz@unb.br (R.P.Z.)

Abstract: This multicenter study aims to assess the impact of public policies (PPs) on the health-related quality of life (HRQoL) of individuals with celiac disease (CD) using the Celiac Disease Questionnaire (CDQ) and PPs for Celiac Disease Score (PPCDS). This cross-sectional exploratory study was conducted in four stages: first, standardizing data from countries using the CDQ; second, analyzing PPs aimed at CD patients; third, statistically examining these data; and fourth, associating HRQoL indicators with corresponding PPs. This study analyzed 15 CDQ assessments from 12 countries from 2007 to 2023. It found that comprehensive PPs positively correlated with HRQoL outcomes (Spearman correlation of 0.358). However, policies specifically targeting gluten-free meals and certification did not significantly improve HRQoL individually, suggesting they may be more effective when implemented together. Additionally, specialized health services did not notably reduce gastrointestinal symptoms, underscoring the necessity for improved patient education to enhance the effectiveness of these services. This study concludes that implementing and rigorously monitoring regulations to support CD patients is crucial for enhancing their HRQoL.

Keywords: regulations; gluten-free; celiac disease public policies; celiac disease questionnaire

1. Introduction

Celiac disease (CD) is a chronic autoimmune enteropathy caused by the consumption of gluten by individuals with a genetic predisposition. Its worldwide prevalence is between 1% and 2% [1–3]. Inflammation of the small intestine and villous atrophy happens to celiacs due to the ingestion of gluten; therefore, the disease treatment consists of a completely gluten-free diet (GFD) [1,2].

The clinical manifestations of CD are classified as classic and non-classic [3,4]. The classic signs and symptoms of the disease are gastrointestinal-related, the most frequent of which are diarrhea, constipation, pain and bloating, flatulence, and weight loss [4,5]. In addition, CD can also present extraintestinal manifestations such as anemia, osteoporosis, recurrent mouth ulcers, chronic fatigue, depression, and dermatitis herpetiform [4,6,7].

Patients often report experiencing symptoms, but there are cases wherein individuals with CD are asymptomatic even when presenting with intestinal mucosal damage [8,9]. The wide range of manifestations and clinical profiles, combined with the complexity of diagnosing this condition, has led to a global underestimation of its prevalence [9–11].

The impact of celiac disease on the well-being of individuals can be significant, affecting various aspects such as physical health, mental well-being, social interactions, and overall daily functioning [3,12]. Several studies used the Celiac Disease Questionnaire (CDQ) by Haüser et al. in 2007, designed to assess health-related quality of life (HRQoL) in patients with celiac disease [13]. Along with determining HRQoL, evaluating the effectiveness of public policies (PPs) on CD outcomes is important since legislation is crucial in providing support and improving the welfare of CD patients [14,15].

Public regulations should cater to individuals' daily challenges with CD, including access to safe dining options and gluten-free products [14,16]. It is crucial to understand the socioeconomic impact of the disease when assessing policy efficacy, as it can lead to financial burdens [14,17]. Policies should aim to provide financial assistance, insurance coverage for gluten-free products, and other forms of support [18].

Different models of financial support for people with CD can be found worldwide. For instance, in Italy and Argentina, the government has established a system through which adults with CD are entitled to an allowance to offset the higher cost of gluten-free foods [16,19], whereas, in Portugal and Australia, a tax deduction is available for people with CD to claim expenses related to gluten-free products [16,20]. These approaches alleviate financial strain and promote the adherence to a strict gluten-free diet [16].

Overall assessment of PPs on CD outcomes requires a multidimensional approach that considers broader societal, economic, and psychological factors affecting affected individuals' HRQoL [21–23]. Recognizing the significance of PPs for CD patients and their influence on quality of life emphasizes the need to evaluate how a country's regulations for CD can directly impact the well-being of individuals with this condition [16,24].

This study aims to assess the correlation between the HRQoL of individuals with CD, as evaluated by the CDQ [13], and the Public Policies for Celiac Disease Score (PPCDS) [25]. By examining these two measures, we can establish the extent to which PPs are linked to enhanced HRQoL for this population.

2. Materials and Methods

2.1. Study Design

This study is a multicenter, cross-sectional exploratory research conducted in four stages: (I) data acquisition and standardization from countries assessing the quality of life (QoL) of individuals with celiac disease (CD) using the CDQ; (II) analysis of public policies targeting people with CD in each participating country, spanning the years of CDQ application and the current study year, employing the PPCDS method; (III) statistical analysis of the gathered data; and (IV) correlation of QoL indicators across studied countries with their respective public policies aimed at the investigated population. A summary of the research process is presented in Figure 1.

To be included in this research, studies must have utilized the complete CDQ instrument for adult patients across various countries. No language or date restrictions were established. Studies that only evaluated children validated the instrument, or did not have openly published data were excluded from the study. Before excluding studies that did not have open data, we attempted contact with the corresponding author via email mentioned in the papers.

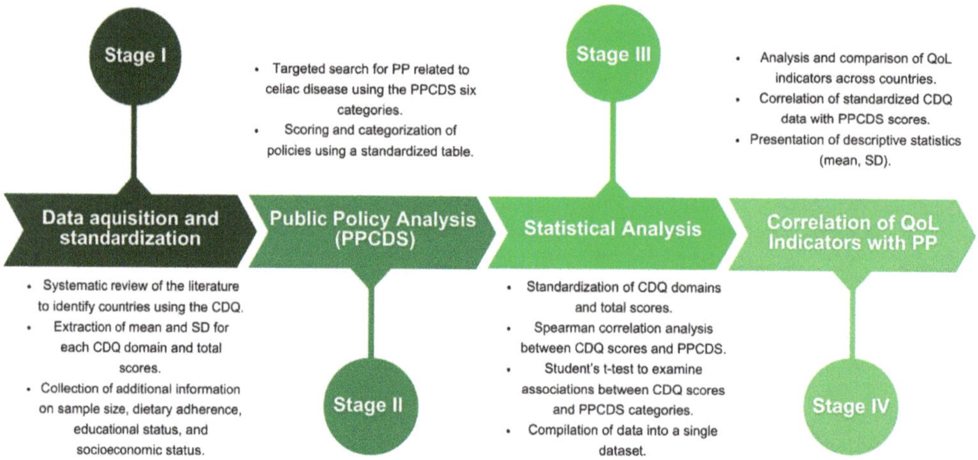

Figure 1. Comprehensive workflow of the multicentric quality of life and public policies for celiac disease research. CDQ: Celiac Disease Questionnaire; SD: standard deviation; PP: public policies; PPCDS: Public Policies for Celiac Disease Score.

2.2. Data Collection and Screening Processes

The process of identifying countries that applied the CDQ instrument involved a systematic review of the published literature using the following terms, their mesh terms, and synonyms: "quality of life" AND ("celiac disease" OR "coeliac disease") AND ("questionnaire" OR "instrument") AND "adults" [26]. Our review was guided by the Preferred Reporting Items for Systematic Reviews and Meta-Analyses protocol, which enabled us to detect studies from different countries that could potentially meet the inclusion criteria [27].

After identifying eligible studies, the researchers extracted the mean and standard deviation of each CDQ domain and total scores for the celiac population in the respective country and year of data collection. Additionally, they gathered information on sample size, dietary adherence, educational status, and socioeconomic status from the CDQ assessment results.

The PPCDS evaluates the level of assistance provided by countries to their celiac populations through the assessment of six categories: the existence of regulations for GF industrial food and GF meals, specialized health service support, food allowance or financial incentives for individuals with celiac disease, gluten-free food certification, and support from celiac disease associations. Each category is scored on a scale from 0 to 1, where 1 represents the presence of relevant policies, and 0 indicates the absence of such policies. The total PPCDS score ranges from 0 to 6, with higher scores indicating more comprehensive and supportive public policies for individuals with celiac disease.

To assess PPs, two investigators conducted a targeted search for each country included in the QoL analysis, examining policy documents, government websites, and published literature on regulations, laws, and programs related to celiac disease from the same year as the instrument application and the current policies. The search strategy was performed using Google Search. It included combined keywords related to gluten-free products, meals, regulations, certifications, labeling, and terms associated with celiac disease, healthcare support, government assistance, and CD societies as proposed by the PPCDS original study [25].

The identified policies were categorized using a standardized table, with each policy marked as either 'Yes' or 'No; for every policy marked as 'Yes", 1 point was allocated. Whenever discrepancies in categorization arose between the two investigators, they discussed and reached a consensus.

For countries with non-English official languages, the searches were conducted in those languages with the assistance of the Google Translator tool. The CDQ scores and PPCDSs were then compiled into a single dataset, with each country represented as a data point.

2.3. Data Standardization and Quantitative Analysis

To allow for comparisons across countries, the CDQ domains and total scores, a 0–100 scale in two studies, were standardized to the instrument's original 28–196 scale, where 196 represents the best possible quality of life [13]. The CDQ is a 28-item instrument that assesses four domains of quality of life: emotion, social, worries, and gastrointestinal. Each domain consists of 7 items scored on a 7-point Likert scale. As a result, the highest possible score for each domain is 49, and the total quality of life score is 196, which represents the sum of all the item scores.

To enable comparability between countries, we used the weighted mean and pooled standard deviation to present the CDQ findings consistently. This weighted comparison was necessary as data from two studies had been calculated for two groups and did not provide a final score [1,19].

After standardizing the CDQ data, we used the Spearman correlation to verify the relationship between the CDQ domains and total scores with the PPCDS. Additionally, a Student's t-test was conducted to examine the strength and direction of the association between the CDQ domain and total scores and the six PPCDS categories. All analyses were performed using IBM SPSS Statistics for Windows [28]. Descriptive statistics, such as the mean and standard deviation, were presented to summarize the statistical analysis of the scores.

3. Results

Of the 21 studies identified through the systematic review, two were excluded for having validated the instrument but not applying it to the population [29,30]; two were excluded due to insufficient data [31,32]; and one was excluded for not thoroughly applying the CDQ instrument [33]. The remaining 15 studies, representing 12 different countries, were included in the final analysis, as they provided the necessary data for analyzing CDQ scores.

3.1. Studies Characteristics

The 15 studies included in the final analysis were conducted between 2007 and 2023 in 12 unique countries: Argentina (n = 1; 6.67%) [34], Australia (n = 1; 6.67%) [35], Brazil (n = 2; 13.33%) [36,37], France (n = 2; 13.33%) [21,38], Germany (n = 1; 6.67%) [13], Iran (n = 1; 6.67%) [39], Italy (n = 2; 13.33%) [3,19], Morocco (n = 1; 6.67%) [40], Portugal (n = 1; 6.67%) [41], Spain (n = 1; 6.67%) [42], Turkey (n = 1; 6.67%) [43] and the United Kingdom (n = 1; 6.67%) [1]. Notably, the dataset includes multiple studies from Brazil (2018 [36] and 2021 [37]), Italy (2011 [19] and 2013 [3]), and France (2014 [38] and 2022 [21]), allowing for an evaluation of temporal trends in these regions.

The geographical distribution of the studies spans five continents, with representation from South America (Argentina, Brazil), Oceania (Australia), Europe (France, Germany, Italy, Portugal, Spain, United Kingdom), Asia (Iran, Turkey), and Africa (Morocco). Most studies were conducted in European countries (n = 8; 53.33%).

In terms of sample characteristics, these studies involved 3982 celiac disease patients, with sample sizes ranging from 45 to 787 participants per study. The average age of the participants ranged from 29.83 to 49.0 years, with a higher proportion of females in all studies.

In some studies, the lack of demographic data on marital status, socioeconomic status, occupational status, education level, and dietary adherence to a gluten-free diet resulted in a subset of participant information being unavailable. This made it impossible to conduct further analysis across all the included studies.

Except for three studies that did not investigate dietary adherence [19,39,42], the celiac patients' adherence to a gluten-free diet ranged from 50% to 100%. The studies used diverse methods to assess self-reported dietary adherence, such as a five-point Likert scale [3,34,36,37,41,43,44], a combination of the CDAT and GDF-S instruments [1], a 10-point visual analog scale [21], three-day food diary as well as self-report adherence [35], and a dichotomous inquiry [40].

Table 1 summarizes the countries' CDQ domain scores and total scores, the PPCDSs, the studies' sample sizes, and publication years. The table was ordered alphabetically and chronologically to optimize visualization in cases with multiple studies for a given country.

Table 1. CDQ scores and PPCDSs by country and year.

	Year	n	PPCDS	CDQ				
				Emotion	Social	Worries	Gastrointestinal	Total
				Mean (SD)	Mean (SD)	Mean (SD)	Mean (SD)	Mean (SD)
Argentina [34]	2020	171	6	26.07 (10.38)	35.80 (9.25)	28.82 (10.11)	33.77 (9.24)	124.14 (32.44)
Australia [35]	2020	45	6	32.90 (0.99)	41.00 (6.12)	39.80 (0.79)	33.00 (0.88)	147.00 (3.31)
Brazil [36]	2018	450	4	27.06 (10.08)	34.67 (7.08)	31.17 (8.54)	35.17 (6.23)	128.06 (27.08)
Brazil [37]	2021	674	4	34.81 (8.42)	25.82 (8.87)	34.86 (10.25)	29.77 (10.75)	125.26 (32.02)
France [38]	2014	211	6	29.55 (9.20)	38.75 (9.91)	34.43 (9.62)	35.98 (8.07)	138.71 (30.91)
France [21]	2022	787	6	33.46 (8.82)	41.44 (8.40)	36.82 (8.82)	38.92 (7.98)	150.64 (20.16)
Germany [44]	2007	446	3	32.30 (8.50)	42.40 (7.10)	37.00 (8.80)	39.30 (7.10)	151.10 (25.20)
Iran [39]	2018	81	1	27.64 (10.81)	29.37 (10.72)	27.11 (10.38)	35.06 (9.76)	119.18 (34.00)
Italy [19]	2011	187	5	32.92 (7.62)	42.09 (6.75)	40.24 (51.34)	39.31 (5.82)	154.53 (20.86)
Italy [3]	2013	171	6	34.00 (8.00)	43.00 (7.00)	40.00 (8.00)	41.00 (7.00)	159.00 (24.00)
Morocco [40]	2022	112	2	26.23 (4.68)	31.76 (9.69)	25.03 (8.36)	34.67 (6.72)	117.73 (24.61)
Portugal [41]	2023	234	6	28.35 (7.60)	23.03 (9.53)	26.77 (8.78)	25.12 (8.81)	103.28 (31.15)
Spain [42]	2022	92	6	27.48 (4.78)	40.23 (5.84)	30.79 (5.72)	32.53 (7.76)	131.03 (24.10)
Turkey [43]	2015	205	4	28.60 (9.00)	34.00 (8.10)	28.00 (8.50)	34.20 (8.30)	124.80 (28.10)
United Kingdom [1]	2021	116	6	34.20 (5.57)	44.10 (6.32)	40.40 (6.78)	37.85 (7.63)	156.55 (21.77)

SD: Standard Deviation; PPCDS: Public Policies for Celiac Disease Score; CDQ: Celiac Disease Questionnaire.

The total CDQ scores varied across countries, reflecting differences in the quality of life among individuals with celiac disease. The highest-scoring countries were Italy, the United Kingdom, and Germany. Italy ranks first and third with the best quality of life among celiac disease patients. The countries with the lowest scores are Iran, Morocco, and Portugal.

For countries that assessed the quality of life at two different time points, Italy and France showed an improvement, going from a score of 154.53 to 159.0 points and from 138.71 to 150.64, respectively. In contrast, a worsening in general QoL was observed in Brazil between 2018 and 2021.

Regarding public policies, Iran, Morocco, and Germany had the lowest scores on the PPCDS scale. Conversely, Italy in 2013, the United Kingdom, Australia, France, Spain, Argentina, and Portugal scored higher on the PPCDS. Details on the scores for each PPCDS category can be found in Table S1 in Supplementary Materials.

3.2. *Public Policies for Celiac Disease Score (PPCDS)*

Figure 2 illustrates variations in the PPCDS across different countries and timelines. Argentina, Australia, France, Italy, and the United Kingdom consistently achieved the highest PPCDS of 6 over multiple years. In contrast, Brazil consistently scored 4 from 2018 to 2024. Germany improved from 3 in 2007 to 6 in 2024, and Turkey's scores increased from 4 in 2015 to 5 in 2024. Although Iran's PPCDS improved from 1 in 2018 to 2 in 2024, it remains categorized in the lower end, similar to Morocco, which maintained a score of 2 over the years. The data also highlight regional disparities, with European and Latin American countries achieving higher PPCDSs than Asian and African nations.

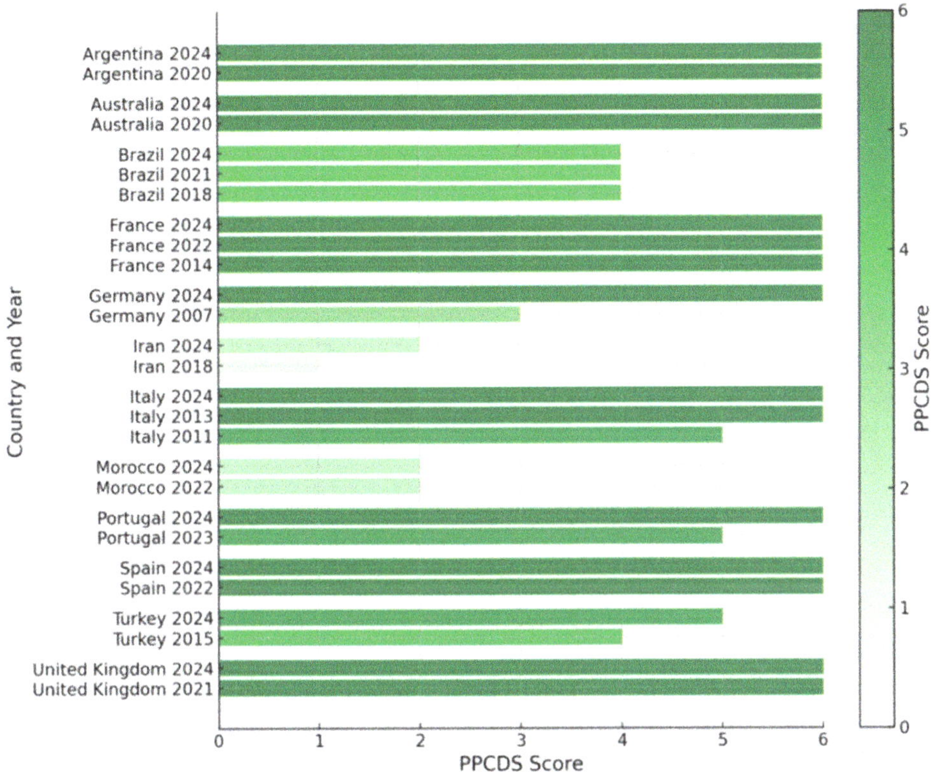

Figure 2. Comparative timeline of PPCDS across countries. PPCDS: Public Policies for Celiac Disease Score.

3.3. Association between HRQoL and PP

Figure 3 presents a spider chart that compares the CDQ domain scores—Emotion, Worries, Gastrointestinal, and Social—across 15 countries and years. Each axis represents one of the four domains, with scores normalized to a common scale from 0 to 49. The chart uses a diverse color palette based on the chromatic circle, ensuring clear differentiation between countries. This visualization allows for a comprehensive comparison of how different countries and years perform across these critical quality-of-life dimensions for individuals with celiac disease. The use of vibrant, non-repetitive colors enhances the chart's readability, making it easier to identify patterns and contrasts in the domain scores across the analyzed countries.

The analysis revealed a positive association between PPCDS and CDQ, with a Spearman correlation score of 0.358. A positive association exists between most PPCDS items and CDQ domains (Table 2). However, the category of meal regulations was associated with reduced scores in the social and gastrointestinal CDQ domains and lower total CDQ scores (Table 2). Additionally, this PPCDS item was not associated with the worries CDQ domain. Furthermore, regulations concerning industrial food products and specialized health services did not show an association with the gastrointestinal CDQ domain. Lastly, gluten-free certification for manufactured meals was not associated with the emotion CDQ domain. Since all countries presented celiac disease associations, the correlation between this PP and CDQ cannot be evaluated.

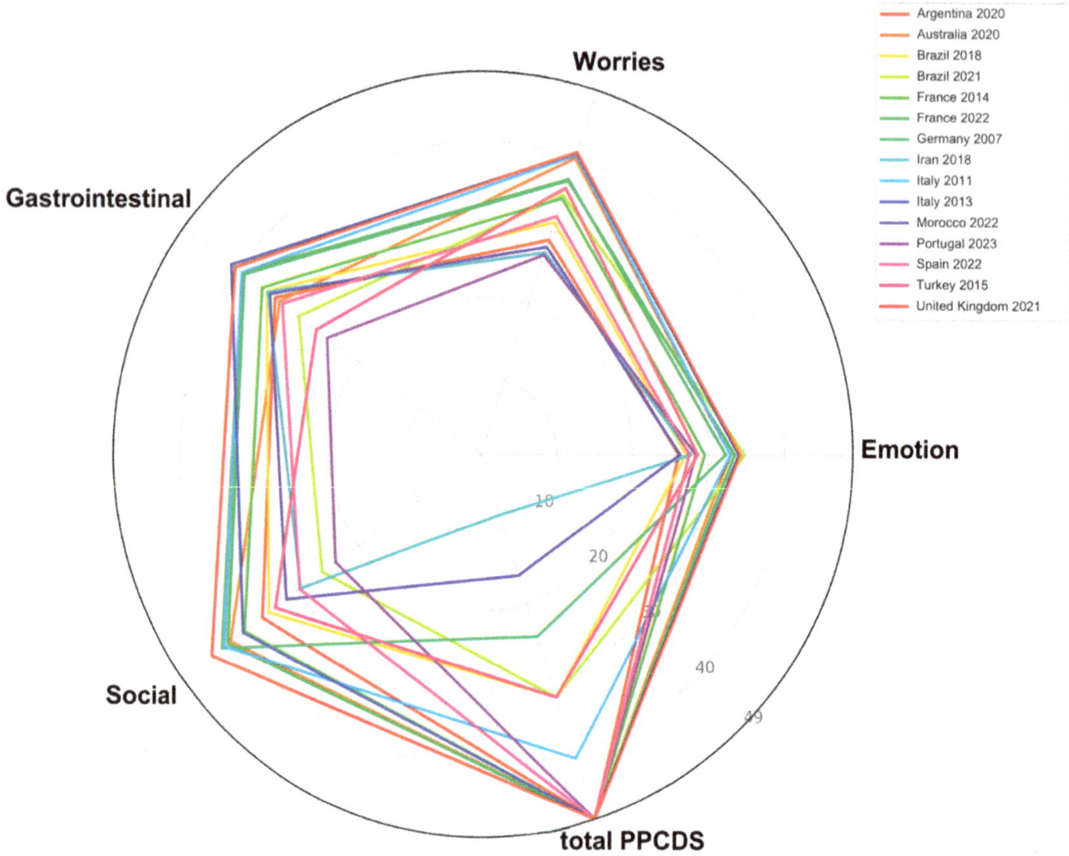

Figure 3. CDQ domain scores and total PPCDSs (normalized) by country and year. CDQ: Celiac Disease Questionnaire; PPCDS: Public Policies for Celiac Disease Score.

Table 2. Relationship between CDQ scores and PPCDS categories.

		Yes	No	p [2]
		Mean (SD) [1]	**Mean (SD)** [1]	
Regulations concerning industrial food products	n	3789	193	
	Emotion	31.54 (8.60)	26.82 (7.85)	0.000
	Social	36.18 (8.11)	30.76 (10.13)	0.000
	Worries	34.54 (14.33)	25.90 (9.26)	0.000
	Gastrointestinal	35.24 (8.20)	34.83 (8.13)	0.496
	Total	137.55 (26.58)	118.34 (28.92)	0.000
Regulations relating to meals	n	2951	1031	
	Emotion	31.54 (8.65)	30.65 (8.32)	0.003
	Social	35.01 (8.34)	38.49 (7.88)	0.000
	Worries	34.26 (8.99)	33.72 (23.24)	0.466
	Gastrointestinal	34.44 (8.48)	37.45 (7.34)	0.000
	Total	135.31 (27.00)	140.36 (25.79)	0.000

Table 2. *Cont.*

		Yes	No	p [2]
		Mean (SD) [1]	**Mean (SD)** [1]	
Specialized health service support	n	3901	81	
	Emotion	31.39 (8.51)	27.64 (10.88)	0.003
	Social	36.05 (8.16)	29.37 (10.79)	0.000
	Worries	34.27 (14.20)	27.11 (10.45)	0.000
	Gastrointestinal	35.23 (8.16)	35.06 (9.82)	0.880
	Total	136.98 (26.52)	119.18 (34.21)	0.000
Food allowance and/or financial incentive	n	2014	1968	
	Emotion	31.58 (8.28)	31.04 (8.84)	0.046
	Social	38.82 (8.28)	32.94 (8.16)	0.000
	Worries	35.31 (17.63)	32.91 (9.27)	0.000
	Gastrointestinal	36.30 (7.82)	34.12 (8.57)	0.000
	Total	142.07 (24.54)	131.03 (28.73)	0.000
Gluten-free certification for manufactured meals	n	2219	1763	
	Emotion	31.31 (8.35)	31.32 (8.86)	0.954
	Social	38.38 (8.26)	32.81 (8.30)	0.000
	Worries	34.63 (16.99)	33.48 (9.44)	0.007
	Gastrointestinal	36.10 (7.87)	34.11 (8.66)	0.000
	Total	140.48 (24.88)	131.75 (29.05)	0.000
Celiac disease Associations [3]	n	3982	0	
	Emotion	31.31 (8.56)	-	-
	Social	35.91 (8.22)	-	-
	Worries	34.12 (14.13)	-	-
	Gastrointestinal	35.22 (8.20)	-	-
	Total	136.61 (26.69)	-	-

[1] Weighted mean and Pooled Standard Deviation; [2] Independent Student *t* test; [3] All countries presented celiac disease associations.

4. Discussion

4.1. Insights on HRQoL Analysis

Both Brazilian studies observed that individuals who followed a strict GFD had higher overall QoL and by domains [36,37]. The same association was observed by the Argentinian [34], French [21,38], Portuguese [41], Turkish [43], British [1], and German [13] studies. Such observations also correlate with the low "worries" subscale scores since they are related to a GFD and, consequently, to regulations for GF products and their enforcement [16,45].

The substantial price gap between GF food and gluten-containing food likely contributes to the observed lower CDQ scores, as affordability concerns can negatively impact the mental well-being and social aspects of individuals with CD, which are directly reflected in the worries and social CDQ domains [46–48]. Studies have emphasized the need for governmental financial aid, as not having access to secure GF products and meals also burdens the health system due to disease advancement [24,49,50].

Strict adherence to the gluten-free diet can enhance physical and physiological well-being. Still, it may also put a strain on mental health and social aspects, as observed in the German celiac disease questionnaire [44]. Individuals may feel insecure about eating out, fear gluten cross-contamination, or be perceived as different for bringing home-cooked gluten-free meals when dining out [23,33]. Access to GF certification could reassure celiacs as it is a form of communication and transparency with consumers [51].

However, according to the latest French celiac disease questionnaire, an essential improvement in health-related quality of life was observed per additional year following the gluten-free diet [21]. The authors believe patients became habituated to managing the restrictive lifelong diet and found comfort in being part of celiac societies, resulting in less reported anxiety and fewer social difficulties the longer they had adhered to the diet [21,33].

Most European countries, with the exception of Portugal, scored higher in the CDQ (Table 1). However, it is essential to note that the assessment of HRQoL of Portuguese celiacs occurred during the COVID-19 pandemic [41]. The two studies that also collected data during the pandemic period were the Spanish and the Brazilian second study [37,42].

Portugal's research obtained general sub-optimal scores, but it should be considered that 44.9% (n = 129) of the study's participants did not follow a strict GFD [41]. Therefore, even though being at home could offer more trust in the secureness of the meal prepared, participants could have fallen into the temptation of eating gluten-containing food with family members, for instance [12,23,41].

According to the study performed in Brazil during the COVID-19 pandemic, Brazilians obtained higher scores in the social and worries domains, which could be related to the fact that 88.57% (n = 597) of the participants adhered to the dietary treatment [37]. The Spanish research also observed a higher score in the social item [42]. As a positive outcome, the pandemic period provided a sense of safety as meals were mainly prepared at home, and celiacs could avoid social events in places with gluten-containing food [37,52].

When analyzing the countries with HRQoL accessed more than once, France and Italy have both bettered their overall scores and subcategories [3,19,21,38]. Brazil obtained an overall score of 1.8 points lower and better in the emotion and worries categories than in the first assessment [36,37]. However, as mentioned, this second CDQ application occurred during the pandemic [37]. Following up on countries' CD HRQoL periodically would be interesting so governments and health professionals can identify opportunities to improve celiac patient support [15,25].

4.2. *Public Policies for Celiac Disease Score (PPCDS)*

As evidenced in Figure 2, the European and Oceanian countries tend to have higher PPCDSs. These continents, alongside North America, have presented an increase in CD diagnoses in recent decades [25,53]. Conversely, the scores indicate that the African and Asian countries maintain relatively lower PPCDSs as in the 2019 assessment [25]. This is likely due to the lack of comprehensive population-based studies in regions such as Africa and Asia, which could explain the lower investment in patient support in those areas compared to other continents [53].

The exception is Turkey, an intercontinental country categorized as an Asian country for analytical purposes by the World Health Organization [54]. Turkey´s one-point improvement in the PPCDS between 2015 and 2024 is due to implementing a financial incentive policy for patients with CD, who are categorized today with a high score [25]. That indicates a national effort to support this population.

Additionally to Turkey, other countries have bettered their PPCDS since the period of the CDQ assessment. In 2007, Germany had a moderate PPCDS of 3 points, which was still higher than Iran and Morocco´s present scores. At the time, Germany presented regulations for gluten-free food products, specialized health services, and celiac society.

Since then, Germany has implemented policies related to partial financial aid through tax deductions for the extra costs associated with gluten-free foods if they exceed a certain percentage of the individual's income. The UK, Spain, Italy, France, Australia, and Portugal already had PPs regarding food allowances or financial support.

The UK expanded the list of items in the GFD prescription provided through the National Health System. Argentina, Italy, and Spain augmented the allowances according to inflation and the cost of GF food and expanded the eligibility criteria. Portugal provided partial subsidies for GF food in 2023 and implemented a new policy giving tax deductions for the additional costs of medically prescribed GF food. Australia adjusted the process of claiming tax deductions for the additional costs of the GFD [20].

It is imperative to highlight that the financial assistance PP is, in all countries included in this study, not available in the whole nation´s territory [48,55]. As celiac disease cases continue to spike, there is an impending need for reevaluating patient care and expanding regulations to ensure patient security [15,56].

Although access to CD diagnostic tools may have increased, healthcare professionals' need for knowledge and the diverse symptoms of this chronic condition still present challenges to suspecting and confirming the diagnosis [57,58]. Therefore, having CD-specialized healthcare is important to minimize delay in diagnosis and reduce exposure to gluten, which impacts QoL and life expectancy [59,60].

Nowadays, all countries included in this research have health centers with pathology-trained professionals. In addition, the records found of these centers were linked to universities, schools, and hospitals in all nations. That suggests that CD knowledge needs to be publicized to already-trained health professionals and beyond the academic sphere [57,58].

Regarding the lowest-scoring countries, as shown in Figure 2, Iran and Morocco´s scores suggest poorer support for individuals with CD in these countries than others. These findings align with [40].

According to the PPCDS data (Figure 2), despite the improvement in Iran´s score, it is still alongside Morocco, the only two countries in this study that lack formal national regulations for gluten-free food labeling. In these countries, industries and restaurants follow general food safety standards focused on quality and safety, but there are no specific gluten-free labeling requirements. This represents food insecurity and elevates worries for individuals with celiac disease [15,56].

Additionally, manufacturers who voluntarily include gluten information to appeal to health-conscious consumers and those with dietary restrictions frequently do not have exclusively gluten-free production [61]. As a result, the imported products certified as gluten-free are the most trustworthy options. Still, they are seen as a luxury since the products are hard to find and have elevated prices, making access to them difficult in Morocco and Iran [18,40].

Since gluten-free products cost more than traditional food items, maintaining a lifelong GFD can be onerous and a significant barrier to treatment adherence [49,62]. As previously documented, the cost disparity between gluten-containing products and gluten-free counterparts varies across countries [14,17]. For example, in Greece, gluten-free products can be 22–334% more expensive in supermarkets and 88–476% in pharmacies [63]. Meanwhile, in Morocco, gluten-free prices can be 115–1309% higher than regular versions [61].

Furthermore, the elevated cost of gluten-free products represents a significant barrier to adhering to the necessary treatment, and the GFD directly impacts the gastrointestinal domains and indirectly affects the emotional and social aspects of health-related quality of life [18,56,62].

4.3. Association between HRQoL and PPs

This study is the first to investigate the relationship between the HRQoL of individuals with CD and the PPs in place for this patient population. The findings reveal a positive correlation between the PPCDSs and the CDQ scores, suggesting that countries with more comprehensive public policies addressing celiac disease tend to have better overall quality of life outcomes for those with this condition.

While most PPCDS components positively correlated with various CDQ domains (Figure 3 and Table 2), indicating broad benefits for celiac patients across different aspects of life, an exception was observed in meal regulations. This specific policy category was associated with lower scores in the social and gastrointestinal domains of the CDQ and the overall CDQ scores.

These meal regulations may not be fully enforced, or their implementation may not effectively address the social and gastrointestinal concerns of individuals with celiac disease. Producing gluten-free meals in professional kitchens that also handle gluten-containing foods can pose significant challenges [64–66]. As a result, individuals with celiac disease often opt to dine in exclusively gluten-free restaurants [62,67,68].

While the meals may be safe, celiacs have reported feeling socially isolated and judged when inviting family members and friends to eat in a 100% gluten-free establishment, which can negatively impact their social experiences [12,23,33]. Hence, having laws to guide GF meal production does not mean that the policies are being followed or that celiac consumers will trust the restaurants; this result suggests that this PP alone will not make people with CD more confident about dining out [23,33,51].

Similarly, the presence of GF certification for manufactured meals did not show a significant positive association in the worries domain of the CDQ, indicating that, while this certification is essential and could be effective, it alone may not be sufficient to alleviate the concerns and fears experienced by individuals with CD [23,33]. Considering that consumers' trust in certifications is related to the perception of credibility in the food production process, the simultaneous implementation of meal regulations and GF certification could be more effective in attenuating concerns about celiacs [51].

Moreover, the availability of specialized health services did not correlate with improvements in the gastrointestinal domain of the CDQ. This absence of association could have been due to the reduced number of specialized health centers in each country. Therefore, celiacs are still attended to, and cared for by health professionals who are not trained in CD [57,58].

4.4. Study Limitations

This study's cross-country comparisons between developed and developing economies with varying public policies may limit the generalizability of its findings to all countries globally. They may not represent continental-level assistance for celiac patients. Additionally, the HRQoL data included only some CDQ assessments made to date, as the researchers could not assess data from three articles that may have met the inclusion criteria despite attempts to contact the authors via email and social media.

Furthermore, the PPCDSs may not fully capture the nuances of how PPs are implemented and enforced across diverse cultural and socioeconomic contexts. Additionally, since some of the policies included in the PPCDS are only regional rather than national, some participants in the CDQ may have access to these policies, which could have diminished the observed association between public policies and quality of life.

5. Conclusions

The findings of this study suggest that PPs designed to address the needs of individuals with CD are associated with better HRQoL outcomes. By highlighting the complex relationship between specific policy domains and various aspects of well-being, this research underscores the importance of a multidimensional approach to policymaking and implementation to support the CD community effectively. Monitoring the enforcement of these regulations, expanding them to all national territories, and educating health professionals to assist celiac patients are necessary steps. Future research should further explore the nuances of policy implementation and additional factors that may influence the QoL for those living with CD. In summary, monitoring the QoL of these individuals over time would provide valuable insights to governments and policymakers.

Supplementary Materials: The following supporting information can be downloaded at https://www.mdpi.com/article/10.3390/nu16172855/s1, Table S1: Public Policies for Celiac Disease Score distribution per country.

Author Contributions: Conceptualization, A.L.F. and R.P.Z.; methodology, A.L.F., R.P.Z. and E.Y.N.; software, E.Y.N.; validation, A.L.F., C.B.P. and R.P.Z.; formal analysis, A.L.F., R.P.Z. and E.Y.N.; investigation, A.L.F.; resources, C.B.P. and R.P.Z.; data curation, A.L.F., E.Y.N., C.C., M.R.-N., M.G., A.A., J.P. and W.H.; writing—original draft preparation, A.L.F.; writing—review and editing, E.Y.N., C.B.P. and R.P.Z.; visualization, C.B.P., C.C., M.R.-N., M.G., A.A., J.P. and W.H.; supervision, R.P.Z.; project administration, R.P.Z.; funding acquisition, C.B.P. and R.P.Z. All authors have read and agreed to the published version of the manuscript.

Funding: This study was partially supported by FAPDF N° 539/2022; and the Brazilian National Council for Scientific and Technological Development (CNPq—N° 302602/2021-6).

Institutional Review Board Statement: Ethical review and approval were waived for this study due to the use of secondary data.

Informed Consent Statement: Not applicable due to the use of secondary data.

Data Availability Statement: Data are contained within the article and Supplementary Materials.

Acknowledgments: Renata Puppin Zandonadi acknowledges the *Fundação de Apoio à Pesquisa do Distrito Federal* (FAP-DF) and the Brazilian National Council for Scientific and Technological Development (CNPq) for their scientific support. The authors acknowledge the financial support of the College of Population Health.

Conflicts of Interest: The authors declare no conflicts of interest.

References

1. Dimidi, E.; Kabir, B.; Singh, J.; Ageridou, A.; Foster, C.; Ciclitira, P.; Dubois, P.; Whelan, K. Predictors of adherence to a gluten-free diet in celiac disease: Do knowledge, attitudes, experiences, symptoms, and quality of life play a role? *Nutrition* **2021**, *90*, 111249. [CrossRef] [PubMed]
2. Mulder, C.J.J.; Van Wanrooij, R.L.J.; Bakker, S.F.; Wierdsma, N.; Bouma, G. Gluten-free diet in gluten-related disorders. *Dig. Dis.* **2013**, *31*, 57–62. [CrossRef]
3. Marchese, A.; Klersy, C.; Biagi, F.; Balduzzi, D.; Bianchi, P.I.; Trotta, L.; Vattiato, C.; Zilli, A.; Rademacher, J.; Andrealli, A.; et al. Quality of life in coeliac patients: Italian validation of a coeliac questionnaire. *Eur. J. Intern. Med.* **2013**, *24*, 87–91. [CrossRef] [PubMed]
4. Caio, G.; Volta, U.; Sapone, A.; Leffler, D.A.; De Giorgio, R.; Catassi, C.; Fasano, A. Celiac disease: A comprehensive current review. *BMC Med.* **2019**, *17*, 142. [CrossRef] [PubMed]
5. Paavola, A.; Kurppa, K.; Ukkola, A.; Collin, P.; Lähdeaho, M.L.; Huhtala, H.; Mäki, M.; Kaukinen, K. Gastrointestinal symptoms and quality of life in screen-detected celiac disease. *Dig. Liver Dis.* **2012**, *44*, 814–818. [CrossRef]
6. Tovoli, F. Clinical and diagnostic aspects of gluten related disorders. *World J. Clin. Cases* **2015**, *3*, 275. [CrossRef]
7. Elli, L.; Branchi, F.; Tomba, C.; Villalta, D.; Norsa, L.; Ferretti, F.; Roncoroni, L.; Bardella, M.T. Diagnosis of gluten related disorders: Celiac disease, wheat allergy and non-celiac gluten sensitivity. *World J. Gastroenterol.* **2015**, *21*, 7110–7119. [CrossRef]
8. Itzlinger, A.; Branchi, F.; Elli, L.; Schumann, M. Gluten-Free Diet in Celiac Disease—Forever and for All? *Nutrients* **2018**, *10*, 1796. [CrossRef]
9. Husby, S.; Koletzko, S.; Korponay-Szabó, I.; Kurppa, K.; Mearin, M.L.; Ribes-Koninckx, C.; Shamir, R.; Troncone, R.; Auricchio, R.; Castillejo, G.; et al. European Society Paediatric Gastroenterology, Hepatology and Nutrition guidelines for diagnosing coeliac disease 2020. *J. Pediatr. Gastroenterol. Nutr.* **2020**, *70*, 141–156. [CrossRef] [PubMed]
10. Singh, P.; Arora, A.; Strand, T.A.; Leffler, D.A.; Catassi, C.; Green, P.H.; Kelly, C.P.; Makharia, G.K. Global Prevalence of Celiac Disease: Systematic Review and Meta-analysis. *Clin. Gastroenterol. Hepatol.* **2018**, *16*, 823–836. [CrossRef]
11. Mustalahti, K.; Catassi, C.; Reunanen, A.; Fabiani, E.; Heier, M.; McMillan, S.; McMillan, S.; Murray, L.; Metzger, M.-H.; Gasparin, M.; et al. The prevalence of celiac disease in Europe: Results of a centralized, international mass screening project. *Ann. Med.* **2010**, *42*, 587–595. [CrossRef]
12. Lee, A.R.; Wolf, R.; Contento, I.; Verdeli, H.; Green, P.H.R.R. Coeliac disease: The association between quality of life and social support network participation. *J. Hum. Nutr. Diet.* **2015**, *29*, 383–390. [CrossRef] [PubMed]
13. Haüser, W.; Gold, J.; Stallmach, A.; Caspary, W.F.; Stein, J. Development and Validation of the Celiac Disease Quality of Life Measure for Adult Patients with Celiac Disease. *J. Clin. Gastroenterol.* **2007**, *41*, 157–166. [CrossRef]
14. Linton, M.J.; Jones, T.; Owen-Smith, A.; Payne, R.A.; Coast, J.; Glynn, J.; Hollingworth, W. Breaking bread: Examining the impact of policy changes in access to state-funded provisions of gluten-free foods in England. *BMC Med.* **2018**, *16*, 119. [CrossRef] [PubMed]
15. Siminiuc, R.; Turcanu, D. Food security of people with celiac disease in the Republic of Moldova through prism of public policies. *Front. Publich Health.* **2022**, *10*, 961827. [CrossRef]
16. Pinto-Sanchez, M.I.; Verdu, E.F.; Gordillo, M.C.; Bai, J.C.; Birch, S.; Moayyedi, P.; Bercik, P. Tax-deductible provisions for gluten-free diet in Canada compared with systems for gluten-free diet coverage available in various countries. *Can. J. Gastroenterol. Hepatol.* **2015**, *29*, 104–110. [CrossRef]
17. Long, K.H.; Wagie, A.E.; Iii, L.J.M.; Lahr, B.D.; Van Dyke, C.T.; Murray, J.A. The economics of coeliac disease: A population-based study. *Aliment. Pharmacol. Ther.* **2010**, *32*, 261–269. [CrossRef] [PubMed]
18. Nadal, J.; Ferreira, S.M.R.; da Costa, I.B.; Schmidt, S.T. The principle of human right to adequate food and celiac disease: Advancements and challenges. *Demetra: Food Nutr. Health* **2013**, *8*, 411–423.
19. Zampieron, A.; Daicampi, C.; Martin, A.; Buja, A. Quality of life in adult celiac disease in a mountain area of Northeast Italy. *Gastroenterol. Nurs.* **2011**, *34*, 313–319. [CrossRef]

20. National Celiac Association. Tax Deductions for Gluten-Free Food. 2024. Available online: https://nationalceliac.org/tax-deductions-for-gluten-free-food/ (accessed on 17 July 2024).
21. Enaud, R.; Tetard, C.; Dupuis, R.; Laharie, D.; Lamireau, T.; Zerbib, F.; Rivière, P.; Shili-Mismoud, S.; Poullenot, F. Compliance with Gluten Free Diet Is Associated with Better Quality of Life in Celiac Disease. *Nutrients* **2022**, *14*, 1210. [CrossRef]
22. Shamir, R.; Heyman, M.B.; Koning, F.; Wijimenga, C.; Gutierrez-Achury, J.; Catassi, C.; Gatti, S.; Fasano, A.; Discepolo, V.; Korponay-Szabó, I.R.; et al. Celiac Disease: Past, Present, and Future Challenges. *J. Pediatr. Gastroenterol. Nutr.* **2014**, *59*, S1. [CrossRef] [PubMed]
23. Bacigalupe, G.; Plocha, A. Celiac is a social disease: Family challenges and strategies. *Fam. Syst. Health* **2015**, *33*, 46–54. [CrossRef]
24. Gatti, S.; Rubio-Tapia, A.; Makharia, G.; Catassi, C. Patient and Community Health Global Burden in a World With More Celiac Disease. *Gastroenterology* **2024**, *167*, 23–33. [CrossRef] [PubMed]
25. Falcomer, A.L.; Luchine, B.A.; Gadelha, H.R.; Szelmenczi, J.R.; Nakano, E.Y.; Farage, P.; Zandonadi, R.P. Worldwide public policies for celiac disease: Are patients well assisted? *Int. J. Public Health* **2020**, *65*, 937–945. [CrossRef]
26. Falcomer, A.L.; de Lima, B.R.; Farage, P.; Fabris, S.; Ritter, R.; Raposo, A.; Teixeira-Lemos, E.; Chaves, C.B.; Zandonadi, R.P. Enhancing life with celiac disease: Unveiling effective tools for assessing health-related quality of life. *Front. Immunol.* **2024**, *15*, 1396589. [CrossRef]
27. Moher, D.; Shamseer, L.; Clarke, M.; Ghersi, D.; Liberati, A.; Petticrew, M.; Shekelle, P.; Stewart, L.A.; PRISMA-P Group. Preferred reporting items for systematic review and meta-analysis protocols (PRISMA-P) 2015 statement. *Syst. Rev.* **2015**, *4*, 1–9. [CrossRef] [PubMed]
28. IBM Corp. *SPSS: Statistical Package for the Social Sciences*; Version 24.0; IBM Corp.: Armonk, NY, USA, 2016.
29. Lobão, C.; Gonçalves, R.; Baltazar, R.M. Desenvolvimento da versão portuguesa do celiac disease questionnaire. *Rev. Int. Cienc. Sociales.* **2013**, *2*, 1–8. [CrossRef]
30. Häuser, W.; Gold, J.; Stein, J.; Caspary, W.F.; Stallmach, A. Health-related quality of life in adult coeliac disease in Germany: Results of a national survey. *Eur. J. Gastroenterol. Hepatol.* **2006**, *18*, 747–753. [CrossRef]
31. Szőcs, H.; Horváth, Z.; Vizin, G. The mediating role of shame in the relationship between stigma and quality of life in patients with celiac disease. *Orv. Hetil.* **2021**, *162*, 1968–1976. [CrossRef]
32. Schiepatti, A.; Maimaris, S.; De Queiros, C.; Archela, M.; Rusca, G.; Costa, S.; Biagi, F. Long-Term Adherence to a Gluten-Free Diet and Quality of Life of Celiac Patients After Transition to an Adult Referral Center. *Dig. Dis. Sci.* **2021**, *67*, 3955–3963. [CrossRef]
33. Zysk, W.; Glabska, D.; Guzek, D.; Głąbska, D.; Guzek, D. Social and Emotional Fears and Worries Influencing the Quality of Life of Female Celiac Disease Patients Following a Gluten-Free Diet. *Nutrients* **2018**, *10*, 1414. [CrossRef]
34. Selleski, N.; Zandonadi, R.P.; Milde, L.B.; Gandolfi, L.; Pratesi, R.; Häuser, W.; Uenishi, R.H.; Nakano, E.Y.; Pratesi, C.B. Evaluation of Quality of Life of Adult Patients with Celiac Disease in Argentina: From Questionnaire Validation to Assessment. *Int. J. Environ. Res. Public Health* **2020**, *17*, 7051. [CrossRef]
35. Harnett, J.E.; Myers, S.P. Quality of life in people with ongoing symptoms of coeliac disease despite adherence to a strict gluten-free diet. *Sci. Rep.* **2020**, *10*, 7–11. [CrossRef]
36. Pratesi, C.B.P.; Häuser, W.; Uenishi, R.H.; Selleski, N.; Nakano, E.Y.; Gandolfi, L.; Pratesi, R.; Zandonadi, R.P. Quality of life of celiac patients in Brazil: Questionnaire translation, cultural adaptation and validation. *Nutrients* **2018**, *10*, 1167. [CrossRef]
37. Falcomer, A.L.; Farage, P.; Pratesi, C.B.; Pratesi, R.; Gandolfi, L.; Nakano, E.Y.; Raposo, A.; Zandonadi, R.P. Health-related quality of life and experiences of brazilian celiac individuals over the course of the sars-cov-2 pandemic. *Nutrients* **2021**, *13*, 1582. [CrossRef]
38. Pouchot, J.; Despujol, C.; Malamut, G.; Ecosse, E.; Coste, J.; Cellier, C. Validation of a French version of the quality of life "celiac disease questionnaire". *PLoS ONE.* **2014**, *9*, e96346. [CrossRef]
39. Barzegar, F.; Pourhoseingholi, M.A.; Rostami-nejad, M.; Gholizadeh, S.; Malekpour, M.R.; Sadeghi, A.; Rostami, K.; Maleki, I.; Shahbazi, S.; Emami, M.H.; et al. Transcultural Adaptation and Validation of Persian Version of Celiac Disease Questionnaire (CDQ); A Specific Questionnaire to Measure Quality of Life of Iranian Patients. *Galen Med. J.* **2018**, *7*, e1106. [CrossRef]
40. Guennouni, M.; Admou, B.; Elkhoudri, N.; Bouchrit, S.; Ait, A.; Bourrahouat, A.; Krati, K.; Hilali, A. Quality of life of Moroccan patients with celiac disease: Arabic translation, cross-cultural adaptation, and validation of the celiac disease questionnaire. *Arab. J. Gastroenterol.* **2022**, *23*, 246–252. [CrossRef]
41. Chaves, C.; Raposo, A.; Zandonadi, R.P.; Nakano, E.Y.; Ramos, F.; Teixeira-Lemos, E. Quality of Life Perception among Portuguese Celiac Patients: A Cross-Sectional Study Using the Celiac Disease Questionnaire (CDQ). *Nutrients* **2023**, *15*, 2051. [CrossRef]
42. Moreno, M.d.L.; Sánchez-Muñoz, D.; Sousa, C. Quality of Life in Teenagers and Adults with Coeliac Disease: From Newly Spanish Coeliac Disease Questionnaire Validation to Assessment in a Population-Based Study. *Front. Nutr.* **2022**, *9*, 887573. [CrossRef]
43. Aksan, A.A.; Mercanligil, S.M.; Häuser, W.; Karaismailoğflu, E. Validation of the Turkish version of the Celiac Disease Questionnaire (CDQ). *Health Qual. Life Outcomes* **2015**, *13*, 1–7. [CrossRef]
44. Häuser, W.; Stallmach, A.; Caspary, W.F.; Stein, J. Predictors of reduced health-related quality of life in adults with coeliac disease. *Aliment. Pharmacol. Ther.* **2007**, *25*, 569–578. [CrossRef] [PubMed]
45. Missbach, B.; Schwingshackl, L.; Billmann, A.; Mystek, A.; Hickelsberger, M.; Bauer, G.; König, J. Gluten-free food database: The nutritional quality and cost of packaged gluten-free foods. *PeerJ* **2015**, *3*, e1337. [CrossRef] [PubMed]

46. Fry, L.; Madden, A.M.; Fallaize, R. An investigation into the nutritional composition and cost of gluten-free versus regular food products in the UK. *J. Hum. Nutr. Diet.* **2018**, *31*, 108–120. [CrossRef]
47. Dietetic Association British. *Policy Statement: Gluten Free Food on Prescription*; Dietetic Association British: Birmingham, UK, 2021.
48. Peters, M.; Crocker, H.; Jenkinson, C.; Violato, M. Withdrawing gluten-free food from prescriptions in England: A mixed-methods study to examine the impact of policy changes on quality of life. *J. Hum. Nutr. Diet.* **2020**, *33*, 453–464. [CrossRef] [PubMed]
49. Mogul, D.; Nakamura, Y.; Seo, J.; Blauvelt, B.; Bridges, J.F.P. The unknown burden and cost of celiac disease in the U.S. *Expert Rev. Pharmacoecon. Outcomes Res.* **2017**, *17*, 181–188. [CrossRef]
50. Whitaker, J.K.H.; West, J.; Holmes, G.K.T.; Logan, R.F.A. Patient perceptions of the burden of coeliac disease and its treatment in the UK. *Aliment. Pharmacol. Ther.* **2009**, *29*, 1131–1136. [CrossRef]
51. Truong, V.A.; Lang, B.; Conroy, D.M. When food governance matters to consumer food choice: Consumer perception of and preference for food quality certifications. *Appetite* **2022**, *168*, 105688. [CrossRef]
52. Kreutz, J.M.; Heynen, L.; Arayess, L.; Vreugdenhil, A.C.E. Celiac Disease and the Gluten Free Diet during the COVID-19 Pandemic: Experiences of Children and Parents. *Medicina* **2023**, *59*, 425. [CrossRef]
53. King, J.A.; Jeong, J.; Underwood, F.E.; Quan, J.; Panaccione, N.; Windsor, J.W.; Coward, S.; deBruyn, J.; Ronksley, P.; Shaheen, A.-A.; et al. Incidence of Celiac Disease is Increasing Over Time: A Systematic Review and Meta-Analysis. *Gastroenterology* **2020**, *115*, 507–525. [CrossRef]
54. World Health Organization (WHO). *Alphabetical List of WHO Member States*; WHO: Geneva, Switzerland, 2019.
55. Ugur, A. Public policies that can be implemented to struggle with celiac disease in Turkey. *J. Econ. Soc. Thought* **2015**, *4*, 411–426.
56. Smeets, S.M.; Kiefte-De Jong, J.C.; Van Der Velde, L.A. Food insecurity and other barriers to adherence to a gluten-free diet in individuals with celiac disease and non-celiac gluten sensitivity in the Netherlands: A mixed-methods study. *J. Clin. Gastroenterol.* **2022**, *56*, 863–868. [CrossRef]
57. Sahin, Y.; Sevinc, E.; Bayrak, N.A.; Varol, F.I.; Akbulut, U.E.; Büкülmez, A. Knowledge regarding celiac disease among healthcare professionals, patients and their caregivers in Turkey. *World J. Gastrointest. Pathophysiol.* **2022**, *13*, 178–185. [CrossRef]
58. Barzegar, F.; Rostami-Nejad, M.; Rostami, K.; Ahmadi, S.; Shalmani, H.M.; Sadeghi, A.; Khani, M.A.; Aldulaimi, D.; Zali, M.R. Lack of health care professional's awareness for management of celiac disease may contribute to under diagnosis of CD. *Gastroenterol. Hepatol. Bed Bench* **2019**, *12*, 203–208.
59. Violato, M.; Gray, A.; Papanicolas, I.; Ouellet, M. Resource use and costs associated with coeliac disease before and after diagnosis in 3,646 cases: Results of a UK primary care database analysis. *PLoS ONE* **2012**, *7*, e41308. [CrossRef]
60. Norström, F.; Lindholm, L.; Sandström, O.; Nordyke, K.; Ivarsson, A. Delay to celiac disease diagnosis and its implications for health-related quality of life. *BMC Gastroenterol.* **2011**, *11*, 118. [CrossRef]
61. Guennouni, M.; El Khoudri, N.; Bourrouhouate, A.; Hilali, A. Availability and cost of gluten-free products in Moroccan supermarkets and e-commerce platforms. *Br. Food J.* **2020**, *124*, 1–13. [CrossRef]
62. MacCulloch, K.; Rashid, M. Factors Affecting Adherence to a Gluten—Free Diet in Adults with Coeliac Disease. *Paediatr. Child Health* **2014**, *19*, 305–309. [CrossRef] [PubMed]
63. Panagiotou, S.; Kontogianni, M.D. The economic burden of gluten-free products and gluten-free diet: A cost estimation analysis in Greece. *J. Hum. Nutr. Dietetics* **2017**, *30*, 746–752. [CrossRef]
64. Falcomer, A.L.; Santos Araújo, L.; Farage, P.; Santos Monteiro, J.; Yoshio Nakano, E.; Puppin Zandonadi, R. Gluten contamination in food services and industry: A systematic review. *Crit. Rev. Food Sci. Nutr.* **2020**, *60*, 479–493. [CrossRef]
65. Farage, P.; Zandonadi, R.P.; Ginani, V.C.; Gandolfi, L.; Nakano, E.Y.; Pratesi, R. Gluten-Free Diet: From Development to Assessment of a Check-List Designed for the Prevention of Gluten Cross-Contamination in Food Services. *Nutrients* **2018**, *10*, 1274. [CrossRef]
66. Miller, K.; McGough, N.; Urwin, H. Catering Gluten-Free When Simultaneously Using Wheat Flour. *J. Food Prot.* **2016**, *79*, 282–287. [CrossRef]
67. De Oliveira, P.M.; Zandonadi, R.P.; Moreira, A.; Cutrim, V.; Nakano, E.Y.; de Queiroz, F.L.N.; Botelho, R.B.A.; Saraiva, A.; Raposo, A. Eating Competence and Aspects Related to a Gluten-Free Diet in Brazilian Adults with Gluten-Related Disorders. *Nutrients* **2022**, *14*, 2815. [CrossRef]
68. Hall, N.J.; Rubin, G.; Charnock, A. Systematic review: Adherence to a gluten-free diet in adult patients with coeliac disease. *Aliment. Pharmacol. Ther.* **2009**, *30*, 315–330. [CrossRef]

MDPI AG
Grosspeteranlage 5
4052 Basel
Switzerland
Tel.: +41 61 683 77 34

Nutrients Editorial Office
E-mail: nutrients@mdpi.com
www.mdpi.com/journal/nutrients

www.ingramcontent.com/pod-product-compliance
Lightning Source LLC
Chambersburg PA
CBHW062101220926
51850CB00010B/2854
* 9 7 8 3 7 2 5 8 6 3 3 4 1 *